BEATING HEROIN

If you have a habit which is giving you hell and ruining your life, reading this book will help you to beat that habit. New advances have now put "light at the end of the tunnel" for heroin users. You can now be helped to beat heroin comparatively easily, if that is what <u>you</u> really want.

If you are a friend, relative or healthcare professional of a heroin user, reading this book will help you to understand why they do what they do and are how they are. That in itself will help them. They desperately need your support. However, remember that nothing can keep an addict off their drug until <u>they</u> themselves really want to get off it.

Heroin addiction has often been a life sentence or a death sentence in the past, but it needn't be any more.

BEATING HEROIN

A SUBSTANTIALLY UPDATED EDITION, JANUARY 2002

CONTENTS

THE "BEATING HEROIN" PROGRAM

GETTING OFF HEROIN; STAYING OFF HEROIN; DISCOVERING AND
CORRECTING THE UNDERLYING
FACTORS THAT LED TO THE ADDICTION, AND KEPT IT GOING.

1. GETTING THE WHOLE PICTURE

Understanding the Whole Person, their Background, their Present
Circumstances, their Desires and Goals and their Unusual/ Disturbed/ Distressed
Chemistry, using **A Systematic Comprehensive Chemical Health Record.**

2. DETOXIFICATION   using

Safe   **Buprenorphine**

Painless
                                    Withdrawal
Easy   Management Medications

Effective
                                    and
Quick

Economical   **Group and Personal Support**

3. MAINTENANCE THERAPY using only as necessary

Naltrexone or Buprenorphine
Serotonin Boosters (SSRIs)
Mood Stabilisers (Usually Epilim)
Stimulant Therapy (Dexamphetamine or Ritalin)
Group and Personal Support

4. UNDERLYING FACTOR DISCOVERY & CORRECTION

Discovery / Correction of the Pre-existing Underlying Factors that led to the
addiction and kept it going, using

The Systematic Comprehensive Chemical Health Record

Shared Consultations

Group Therapy

Individual, Couples and Family Counselling

Psychiatric and Psychological Assessment and Treatment where necessary

Long Term Specialised Groups & Other Treatments as Appropriate

FREEDOM FROM SUBSTANCE ABUSE AND ADDICTION

We will never rid Our People   or   Our Families and Communities   or   Our Economy from the curse of impoverishing, shattering, tormenting and sometimes fatal, drug addictions and from the curse of corrupting, disrupting, ruthless and sometimes rich and powerful drug dealers

until we grasp the fact that substance abuse and addiction, are about some people having unusual/disturbed/distressing chemistry

which causes these individuals suffering, and disturbed function/performance, sufficient to cause them to seek to relieve their distress, and to change their function/performance, by taking drugs.

We must grasp the fact that it is of fundamental importance for us to learn to substantially correct addiction prone people's underlying unusual/disturbed/distressing chemistry.
It is not enough for us to detox and return addicts to how they were before their addiction began.

We must accurately define the nature and causes of the particular underlying chemical problems, in each different substance abuse prone or addicted person and have a range of treatments/systems/facilities and specially trained and empowered healthcarers, that enables quick and effective correction of the particular chemical problems in particular individuals

through vigorous simultaneous approaches, from many different angles, and in many different ways, so that each of these individual's chemical functioning, is quickly improved to a level which relieves their distress and dysfunction sufficiently to allow each of these individuals to desire to be free and to be freed and to stay free, from the need to manipulate their chemistry with drugs.

The great bottleneck in the management of our drug problems in the year 2001, is the shortage of health carers capable of diagnosing all the people with ADD who have become cannabis, speed or narcotic addicts because of their unusual and distressing ADD chemistry; together with the excessive, unnecessary difficulties in gaining permission to prescribe dexamphetamine or ritalin, which are by far the most effective initial treatment for ADD and which should be available through every properly staffed and provisioned detox clinic.

At present the vast majority of drug and alcohol workers are not trained to diagnose the commonest cause of addiction which is ADD; and 98% of doctors are not allowed to prescribe the most necessary treatment for that commonest cause.

CHEMICALS AND CHEMICALLY DISTURBED PEOPLE

SUBSTANCES WHICH CHEMICALLY UNUSUAL / DISTURBED / DISTRESSED PEOPLE FREQUENTLY TURN TO, BUT WHICH CAN BE VERY DESTABILISING & DESTRUCTIVE, ARE:

ALTERNATIVE SUBSTANCES, WHICH IN VARYING AMOUNTS & COMBINATIONS, WILL OFTEN STABILISE & SATISFY CHEMICALLY UNUSUAL/ DISTURBED/ DISTRESSED PEOPLE, WITHOUT LEADING TO POVERTY OR HEALTH, SOCIAL OR LEGAL PROBLEMS, & WHICH ARE COMPATIBLE WITH WORK OR STUDY, ARE:

Excessive Caffeine

Nicotine

Excessive Alcohol

Cannabis

Petrol, Glue & Solvent sniffing

LSD

Benzodiazepines, more than 5 tablets per week

Rohypnol

Ecstasy

Street Amphetamines

Narcotics

Cocaine

Buprenorphine – a mild narcotic with powerful blocking effects that keep out more powerful, more dangerous narcotics

Dexamphetamine & Ritalin, freer availability of which would drastically reduce the dangerous street amphetamines trade and usage

Serotonin Boosters (SSRIs) e.g., Efexor XR, Avanza and Cipramil

Tricyclic Antidepressants eg. Doxepin & amitryptiline (prescribed & dispensed in safe amounts), mainly for sleep & sedation, as a highly preferable alternative to Benzodiazepines (benzos)

The Mood Stabilisers, Sodium Valproate (Epilim), Lithium, Clonazepam and Carbamazepine (Tegretol)

The Major Tranquillizers/Antipsychotics Zyprexa & Pericyazine

Benzodiazepines – occasionally. They are much better avoided – in 90% of cases. Temazepam is the safest and should usually be prescribed with only eight tablets (no capsules) to be dispensed every 5 days, or better still, only 5 tablets every eight days

Once a person has become more stable and has resumed a more normal lifestyle, with the help of some of these <u>Alternative</u>, less dangerous <u>Substances</u>, they will often find that their body chemistry becomes more comfortable.
Gradual weaning from the <u>Alternative Substances</u> is then possible, depending on the extent of any remaining undiscovered, untreated Preexisting Underlying Factors, and the severity and duration of the previous Substance Abuse.

Sometimes, as the Alternative Substances are reduced, there will be a deterioration in the person's condition. For the time being, the dose should then be put back up to the last satisfactory level. These Alternative Substances should never be reduced quickly, or stopped suddenly. The risk in coming off these safe or less damaging alternative substances, is that there may be a recurrence of the chemically based distress and then a craving for and a relapse to the original More Severely Damaging Substances. Reducing the Alternative Substances too fast often results in it taking longer for people to become drug free, because of relapses.

Substance abusers and addicts often have a tendency to make decisions and do things quickly or suddenly. They may be unrealistically anxious to be rapidly and completely substance free. They often have to learn the hard way, through relapses, the dangers of reducing their medicines too soon or too quickly. If they do slip they should be encouraged to just promptly go back to the Alternative Substances again, for a little longer.

It is almost always essential for long term recovery from addiction, for careful psychological, social or psychiatric assessments to be made and for adequate one to one counselling and group therapy to take place. The sooner this is done the sooner the Alternative Substances or medicines can be stopped. If the medicines are stopped before the psychosocial work is done, then relapse to addiction is likely to occur.

Normalisation or stabilisation of brain wave patterns and chemical flows, through a course of EEG Biofeedback, is a very promising new way of facilitating chemical and mental health and reducing the length of time

Alternative Substances or maintenance medications are needed.

WHAT IS HEROIN?

Heroin is an opium poppy derivative which has very strong effects on the brain.

It is very strong medicine, but with horrible side effects if addiction occurs, which it often rapidly does. Some people are particularly prone to narcotic addiction.

Heroin relieves physical pain and mental discomfort or suffering and it may give a high. It sometimes makes people drowsy, but may also give the strength to do things that otherwise could not be done.

However heroin has such serious side effects that these side effects always far outweigh any benefits and cause much more suffering than did any problems for which the heroin was taken in the first place. The brief patches of relief or elation it gives, are outweighed one hundred fold by the suffering that follows.

Heroin is rapidly and strongly addictive, with consequent hanging out pain. It is financially devastating and damaging to relationships, families and employment. It leads to contact with the criminal world, crime and often to poverty, bankruptcy, divorce, serious health problems & jail.

To be effective the Treatment of Heroin Addiction must address two areas.

1. The Addiction.

2. The Discovery and the Resolution of The Pre-existing Underlying Factors which led to the addiction in the first place and then kept it going. These factors exist in every case.

If the second area is not going to be tackled vigorously, tackling the first area may lead to as many problems as it solves and may not be wise in some cases.

"HEROIN IS SUGAR COATED HELL"

PRE-EXISTING UNDERLYING FACTORS WHICH CAN LEAD TO HEROIN ADDICTION

Heroin addiction and dependence on other narcotics, or substances such as alcohol, cannabis, amphetamines, cocaine and prescribed medications, are almost never primary conditions. They are nearly always secondary conditions, the result of Pre-existing, Underlying, physical, chemical, mental or social problems.

To talk about alcoholism or heroin addiction and the treatment of alcoholism or heroin addiction, without discussing the Pre-existing Underlying Factors that lead to the abuse of these substances, is very common and totally counterproductive. Success in detoxification is much less likely, and relapse back to substance abuse is much more likely, if the Underlying Factors are not discovered and successfully treated. Substance abuse is like any other health problem – its treatment must be determined by the diagnosis. "Heroin Addiction" is not a complete diagnosis. The Pre-existing Underlying Factors/ Conditions are the main diagnosis. They must be discovered so that they can then be treated appropriately. To be effective, the diagnosis of the Underlying Factors and their treatment, must commence at the same time as the assessment and treatment of the addiction.

Seeing 50 or 60 patients a week in my drug and alcohol practice has led me to the conclusion that The Pre-existing Underlying Factors/ Conditions in the vast majority of heroin addicts, alcoholics, amphetamine, cannabis and prescribed medication abusers, in order of frequency, are:

1. **ADD** (Attention Deficit Disorder) is very common.

2. **Unresolved Traumas and Stresses** are very common. e.g. verbal, physical or sexual abuse in childhood, deaths in the family, family breakdowns, horrendous motor vehicle accidents, immigration, moving house and school too often, war experiences, serious illness etc.

3. **Depression** is very common. Manic Depressive (Bipolar) Disorder.

4. **Anxiety** and Panic Disorders are common. Social Phobia and Agoraphobia

5. **Insomnia and other Sleep Disorders**.

6. **Chronic Pain** Including Headache, Painful Diseases (eg Pancreatitis), Motor Vehicle, Industrial and Sporting Accident Induced Pain.

7. **Intolerable Circumstances** in the present (violence, relationship breakdowns, financial disasters, accidents, unemployment, problems in the family, at school or at work and collisions with the law, including court appearances and jail.)

8. Being often in a **Drug Environment** in which there is exposure to people using drugs, easy availability of drugs, exposure to drug pushers, peer pressure or an addicted partner.

9. **Lack of Purpose** in life, boredom.

10. **An Unstructured Life**, lack of boundaries, responsibilities or work.

11. **Social Slackness** or weakness in the individual, the family or the environment he grew up in. Self-indulgent people who will try anything or do anything that might gratify them, regardless of possible consequences. This is an uncommon cause of addiction, even though it is often thought to be the main cause.

12. **Serious Sexual Problems**, including Sexual Identity Conflict and the fear of "coming out".

G.D. male, 44 years

I first attended Dr Beck's Chemical Health Centre because of an addiction which arose from being given morphine whilst waiting for surgery. Before seeing Dr Beck I had been switched from morphine to 30 mg of methadone a day. I was also on eight cones of marijuana, 45 mgm of Avanza, Valium and twenty cigarettes each day. I had been chronically depressed most of my life. I took narcotics from the age of fourteen to twenty. I had smoked cannabis heavily on and off for many years. I gave it up from time to time, but always became severely depressed and suicidal again within a few months and went back to the cannabis. I had been on at least six different antidepressants over the years, but none of them seemed to work for me.

I was kicked out of the family home at the age of fourteen for verbal abuse of my mother and was always bullied and disliked at school. I suffered sexual abuse at 11 years of age and in my teens. I always had trouble with sleeping. I often suffered from anxiety, panic attacks, social phobia, severe agitation, violent outbursts and rage. I was diagnosed as ADD, Manic Depressive Disorder or Post Traumatic Stress Disorder by various doctors and psychiatrists over the years. Dexamphetamine prescribed for ADD made me violent but I probably took too much of it, which I tended to do with everything. I had various jobs in the media including important positions at times, but always got fired sooner or later. I attempted suicide five times over a period of many years. I drank a bottle of Scotch every night for 25 years.

Dr Beck considered that my most basic problems were my chronic depression, ADD and the many severe traumas that I had suffered. Together these had caused me to seek relief through polydrug use and this gave me some short term benefits, but overall it increased and aggravated my problems substantially. My main desire when I first went to Dr Beck, was to be free of cannabis and methadone permanently.

Dr Beck started me on buprenorphine and Epilim on the first day. I was able to stop the methadone and my use of marijuana reduced substantially quite quickly. There was an immediate improvement in my general condition. I have not needed methadone or illicit narcotics since.

However my ADD symptoms came back to haunt me, when the methadone and cannabis were stopped and my sleeping difficulties were terrible. I sometimes didn't sleep at all, my depression remained and I was often in tears. I had discussions with Dr Beck and with my psychiatrist about the various antidepressants I had tried without success. Dr Beck put me on an old fashioned antidepressant called Doxepin in the early evening, to help with sleep. My psychiatrist reviewed all the antidepressants I had taken over the years and found that Efexor XR had helped me a little more than the others. I improved greatly with a period on buprenorphine 8 mgm, Doxepin 100 mg in the early evening, 150 mg of Efexor XR in the evening, 500 mg of Epilim in the morning and 1000 mg in the evening and small doses of dexamphetamine in the morning. After stabilizing on these medications and psychological counselling, I am now doing well on a much reduced and simplified medication regime.

I have now had no methadone or illicit narcotics for five months. I don't use cannabis or alcohol at all. I have been able to establish a new home and to improve my relationship with my partner. Despite having a serious car accident recently (not my fault), I am cheerful and have a sense of humour for the first time for many years. I have recently applied for a job for the first time in six years.

Dr Beck tells me that I will need to continue on with the Doxepin, Efexor XR and dexamphetamine in reduced doses for at least a couple of years, until I have broken right out of the vicious cycles which I have been in for most of my forty-four years and have become more permanently chemically, emotionally and socially stabilised. I think he is right when he tells me that the main problems that led to my addictions were brain chemistry abnormalities, due to ADD, multiple psychosocial traumas and chronic depression. These chemical abnormalities are presently being corrected artificially by my medicines, but we believe that now my life has improved so much, my own chemical systems have started to heal and do their job better and my need for medicines will decrease. I am willing to accept that I may need some medicine for two to five years. I also know that I will need ongoing counselling, perhaps for years, but I happily accept that as I find it helps me to grow and to progress. Although therapy is sometimes hard, at other times it is really enjoyable and gratifying. Good therapy is a real treat for someone who has had my problems.

Dr Beck tells me that EEG Biofeedback would almost certainly speed things up and be more of a permanent cure for me, but I can't afford it yet and he can't yet afford to provide that equipment for the clinic, where he hopes in future to provide EEG Biofeedback at a discounted fee for people recovering from addiction problems.

Looking back, I now consider that the most important things in recovering from addiction are understanding and persistence. You need to discover and understand your underlying problems; and then if one medicine doesn't work, after a reasonable trial, you just have to move on to try others. Sooner or later you find the medications that work for you; and you just persist in chipping away, a bit at a time, with the counselling and psychotherapy; and then you get better in fits and starts and heal and escape from your nightmare. At least that is what is happening for me in Dr Beck's Chemical Health Centre.

A SIMPLE SCHEME FOR BEATING HEROIN WHICH ONLY WORKS IN EARLY, MILD CASES

The Simplest Form Of Detoxification From Heroin Is:

i   You stop pushing heroin into your body.

ii Your body continues, as usual, to break down and excrete any heroin it contains, until there is none left.

iii You hang out through the withdrawal period, until all the heroin is gone.

iv You live happily ever after without heroin.

This Simple Strategy Doesn't Very Often Work. The Problems Are:

i   You probably won't have the motivation, or the determination to successfully complete the strategy, if your Preexisting, Underlying Addiction Factors aren't being discovered and dealt with.

ii The withdrawal symptoms may be too much for you to bear and you may lapse back to using heroin again on the second or third day.

iii Even if you do succeed in getting off heroin, the craving persists and there is a 90% chance that you will go back to it again, usually because of this craving and the Preexisting Underlying Factors, if they haven't been dealt with.

iv Sometimes people get through to the 3rd or 4th day, then can't cope any longer and use their previous dose of heroin again. Because they have lost some of their tolerance in that 3 or 4 days of not using, this dose may cause them to OD, if it is taken whilst on benzos or when drunk.

Trying to get off heroin is a dangerous time and addicts need informed support and usually, more sophisticated methods.

A BRIEF COMPARISON OF DETOXIFICATION METHODS

In **Home Detoxification**, the addict simply stops his drug of addiction and then has to get through four or five days of very painful and distressing withdrawal symptoms. Even in a hospital or a special detox unit, there may be great suffering, a high failure rate and some risk of OD if it fails.

In **Rapid Detox, substantial intravenous** injections of narcan are used to **rapidly** block or displace **all** residual heroin in your body, whilst clonidine and four or more other **Withdrawal Management Medications**, are **injected intravenously** to minimize the withdrawal symptoms. The withdrawal symptoms are severe, because there is such a rapid reduction in the heroin levels, due to the **substantial intravenous** narcan injections; especially if you haven't stopped or substantially reduced your heroin intake in the previous three days. This means that high doses of **Withdrawal Management Medications intravenously** are needed; (clonidine, sedatives, vomiting, diarrhoea, cramp and painkilling medications) and they cause their own problems.

The **Rapid Withdrawal,** together with all the **Withdrawal Management Medications** injected straight into the blood stream, may make you very uncomfortable and quite disturbed and dependant on others to care for you for a few hours or days. Dehydration and the need for a drip or hospitalization is possible.

There are advantages with a new alternative, **Incremental (Stepped) Rapid Detoxification**, in which **very small** doses of Narcan (Naloxone) subcutaneously and naltrexone orally, are given every hour or so, together with reduced **Withdrawal Management Medications, mostly orally**, as necessary. These **smaller**, more tolerable bites of Rapid Detox every hour or so, given by the **slower oral** and **subcutaneous routes, get rid of the heroin more quickly and surely than simple Home Detoxification,** but **more slowly, a bit at a time**, than with intravenous **Rapid Detoxification**. If the steps turn out to have been too fast and excessive withdrawal symptoms develop, the situation can be controlled quickly by sucking Buprenorphine tablets. There is less need for **Withdrawal Management Medications**, staff and facilities. There is less drama, trauma and cost, than with Rapid Detox. The patient is alert and in direct consultation with his doctor, with ongoing assessment, problem solving and support until the situation has been resolved. It is possible to be detoxed and stabilized on Naltrexone Maintenance Therapy with 2 to 4 small manageable bites. However it does involve attending the clinic for 2 to 3 hours on 2 or 3 successive days.

The **Best Detox Option is S.P.E.E.Q.E. (Safe, Painless, Easy, Effective, Quick, and Economical) Detoxification.** All narcotics are reduced or stopped and repeated small doses of Buprenorphine are sucked under the tongue as necessary, as soon as the patient starts to feel withdrawal symptoms. Three days after the last heroin, 5 days after the last morphine or 21 days after the last methadone, very small test doses of narcan may be given subcutaneously. Very small test doses of naltrexone are given after each dose of narcan. If a withdrawal reaction occurs, the narcan and naltrexone are stopped, as this reaction means the patient is not yet clean. More Buprenorphine tablets are then sucked and additional time is allowed, so that the narcotics of addiction can be further broken down and excreted by natural body processes. The narcan and naltrexone are then recommenced, proceeding more slowly than before. At Western Australian prices the amount of Buprenorphine needed each day will cost approximately 10% as much as the heroin has been costing. That is, someone spending $100 per day on heroin will need to spend about $10 per day on Buprenorphine. (From August 2001 the Australian Government has subsidised Buprenorphine, reducing the cost to a maximum of $A4 per day, regardless of the daily amount needed. This makes it better for most people to continue on with the buprenorphine for a few weeks or months until all the Pre-existing, Underlying Factors have been discovered and corrected; **in this case narcan and naltrexone are no longer needed – I very seldom use them now.)**

THE GREAT BUPRENORPHINE BREAKTHROUGH

A great breakthrough has recently occurred for narcotic addicts in Western Australia. Buprenorphine has become available for narcotic detoxification, and as a maintenance therapy alternative to Methadone. Buprenorphine was previously available in this country for treating pain, but not for treating addiction since 1984, when it became severely regulated. It has been available for treating narcotic addiction in France for 5 or 6 years where it's use has been very successful. Its use in narcotic addiction is now rapidly spreading throughout the world.

Buprenorphine is a man made narcotic which is usually compatible with naltrexone, and is the least addictive moderately powerful narcotic there is. It is both a moderate agonist and a powerful antagonist (blocker) of the opioid nerve receptors. This means that it both provides moderate narcotic effect, and strongly blocks the craving for and effects of other narcotics, if the appropriate dose is given.

The step from heroin to being clean, which is usually so difficult, distressing and potentially dangerous, can now be painless, easy, cheap and quite safe.

The heroin is simply stopped and as soon as hanging out begins, it is relieved by sucking Buprenorphine tablets under the tongue as necessary, starting with 1 to 2 mgms every half hour, to prevent the occasional side effects of nausea and headache. After three or four days, the breakdown and excretion of all heroin by natural body chemical processes has usually occurred and the addict is clean. If necessary this may be confirmed with a tiny (40mcg) dose of narcan, given subcutaneously.

I now usually keep the patients on buprenorphine in reducing doses until the Pre-existing, Underlying Causes have been discovered and corrected, when we gradually wean off the buprenorphine. Alternatively, after 5 days, Naltrexone can be commenced, starting with very small doses crushed up in water or cordial. The sucking of Buprenorphine is stopped when the gradual introduction of naltrexone is commenced. The Buprenorphine is then broken down and excreted by natural body processes, with minimal discomfort, over the next few days. The naltrexone is continued as a maintenance blocker for as long as the healthcarers consider it necessary. It suppresses any craving, so that the addict doesn't usually even think about heroin. If for any reason the addict does use again, there will be no result, as long as he has taken his naltrexone. Naltrexone blocks the heroin from reaching the nerve endings and therefore from giving a result. It stops the ex addict from becoming addicted again. Naltrexone has debilitating side effects in some people, and may not be needed for long if a vigorous and successful effort is made to discover and correct all the Pre-existing Underlying Factors/ Conditions that led to and perpetuated the patient's addiction.

In a small number of people with serious problems, Buprenorphine (or Naltrexone) may have to be continued for a longer period as maintenance therapy, just as Methadone has been used in the past. It is vastly superior to heroin as maintenance therapy, almost always superior to Methadone and superior to morphine, probably making the idea of trialing or legalizing heroin or morphine as maintenance therapy, unnecessary.

K.B. female, 31 years

I am a single parent living on social security payments. I consulted Dr Beck because of a $50 a day heroin habit which I had had for five weeks and which I couldn't afford. At the time I was also smoking thirty cigarettes a day which I also couldn't afford. I had previously had an intravenous oxycontin habit for which I had rapid detoxification and naltrexone. After a year I felt bad again, stopped the naltrexone, and went on to heroin. I had been working with a psychologist with considerable benefit, but he suddenly became unavailable to me and this was a critical let down that made me vulnerable again.

Dr Beck and Wendy, the counsellor/ psychologist, diagnosed my problems as being instability, anxiety and depression, related to the early break up of my parents' marriage, the fact that my mother had moved so often that I had attended thirteen different schools, had ten different homes and many different step-fathers, one of whom sexually abused me. They did not think that I had ADD. Amphetamines made me very anxious rather than calming and focusing me.

I attended the Shared Consultations conducted by Dr Beck, was given information to read, a copy of the first edition of Dr Beck's Beating Heroin book, had regular One to One Counselling with Wendy, and was put on Cipramil and buprenorphine. Doxepin was later added in the early evenings, to help me sleep.

I was hanging out at the first Shared Consultation and Dr Beck gave me an 8mgm buprenorphine tablet to suck, one quarter at a time, so that I was much improved before I even left the first Shared Consultation. I have not used illicit narcotics since that time, am much calmer and happier, sleeping well and am benefiting from the Shared Consultations and the counselling. Dr Beck thinks I will need to go on with the One to One Counselling or Group Therapy for at least a year, but that I will be able to stop the medication sooner than that if I am able to resolve my Preexisting, Underlying Issues to a sufficient degree. This holistic approach seems to be working well for me. I just didn't have enough information, counselling and support before.

S.P.E.E.Q.E. DETOXIFICATION

(i)   Get the patient to state and repeat several times, whether or not they truly wish to get off and stay off Narcotics and leave the drug world. Listen carefully to the voice volumes and tones and observe carefully the facial expressions. Try to determine their real desires and intentions from this body language. Get them to reinforce their intention by repeating it several times in a louder and louder voice.

(ii) If you feel that there is a reasonable chance that they do wish to get off and to stay off Narcotics, then ask them to stop their Narcotics and immediately give them one mgm of Buprenorphine to suck under the tongue. Give them another 2mgms to suck half an hour later, if the first 1mgm causes no problems. (See special notes on withdrawal from Methadone under item (x) below as withdrawal from Methadone is more complicated and slower). If given too large a starting dose vomiting, headache, precipitated withdrawal and respiratory distress may very occasionally occur. Buprenorphine is strong medicine and the first few doses of a strong medicine should nearly always be small, to detect sensitivities or side effects, even though these are uncommon with Buprenorphine.

If you have serious doubts about the clarity or certainty of their desire to give up Narcotics, discuss with them the need for clarity of desire and determination if they are to succeed. Even if motivation is in doubt, it is usually best to proceed, as an abortive first attempt is likely to promote success later on.

(iii) Ask the patient to take no more Narcotics till you see them again, supply them with a further 2 to 8 mgms to suck that evening and supply them with Withdrawal Management Medications as you think necessary (Clonidine 50– 75mgms 4 hourly, Maxalon, Imodium, Vioxx or Surgam, Sleepers, Tranquillizers, Quinine Bisulphate and Buscopan. Very few Withdrawal Management Medications are needed with this technique).

(iv) The patient should then go home and be cared for by a friend, relative or volunteer and come back for review the next day.

(v)   At review the next day, check for vomiting, headaches, excessive drowsiness, dehydration, insomnia, any other withdrawal symptoms, signs of intoxification with other drugs and the patient's general condition. Nausea and vomiting should be treated with metaclopramide, promethazine, haloperidel, or zofran wafers. If there are no undue problems (which is usually the case) then an 8mgm tablet can be supplied or prescribed, to be taken over the next 24 hours. It should be sucked in quarters or halves, as needed and tolerated.

If there have been or still are side effects or an unacceptably strong withdrawal reaction, go back to reduced doses of the drug of addiction until everything settles down. Then recommence the Buprenorphine treatment at lower doses and increase steadily, according to responses, up to a maximum daily dose of 16mgm. Some overlap of the drug of addiction and the buprenorphine may be needed at times. As Buprenorphine has a very long half life and gradually accumulates in the body, the daily intake can sometimes be reduced after a few days.

(vi) The advantage of the smaller 0.2mgm tablets is that the Buprenorphine can more easily be introduced in smaller amounts and increased more gradually, reducing the chances of Precipitated Withdrawal with Methadone, or of the nausea and vomiting a few patients get with a new narcotic. The advantage of the larger 8mgm tablets is that they are one tenth the cost per mgm of the medication. Of course the larger tablets can easily be cut or broken into halves, quarters or eighths and this is often satisfactory. It is usually best to start with 8mgm tablets. Any intolerance which may very occasionally occur can then usually be overcome by switching to the 0.2 mgm strength tablets and then slowly working back up to the 8mgm tablets again.

If you give the patient too large a prescription for tablets on the first or second day, they often won't come back for review and fine tuning till they have used them all, run out, think they have beaten their addiction and are back in trouble again. Some authorities insist that each dose be administered directly to the patient by a pharmacist. Whilst there are diversion and other not very strong arguments in favour of this policy, it greatly reduces flexibility and success in treating patients in the first place.

(vii) The patient should be seen very often until they have had no heroin or similar Narcotic for 5 days. At that point, they can continue to suck Buprenorphine as necessary, or they can be given very small doses of Naloxone (Narcan) and Naltrexone (Revia). The needle of a 100 unit insulin syringe containing 120mcg of Narcan in 30 units is pushed into the subcutaneous tissues of the upper outer arm and the syringe is strapped in place firmly with adhesive tape. 10 units of the mixture containing 40mcg of Narcan is then injected subcutaneously.

A mixture of 1 crushed Naltrexone tablet in 2 litres of water, cordial or juice (50mgm in 2000mls) is prepared. Five minutes after receiving the Narcan, 40mls of this mixture, well shaken, (1mgm of Naltrexone) is given to the patient to drink. The patient with friend, relative, nurse or volunteer is allowed to rest and watch T.V., have a cup of tea, sit in the fresh air, go for a walk etc.

(viii) If the Naltrexone Option is chosen – and we seldom use it now - after about 45 minutes they are checked for withdrawal symptoms (yawning, sneezing, watering eyes or nose, goose bumps, arm leg or back aches, hot & cold sweats, gut cramps, diarrhea or vomiting). If there is no reaction at all, then they are probably Opiate free and ready for Naltrexone. Give them a further 20 units or 80mcg of Narcan and then 40mls (1 mgm) of Naltrexone mixture 5 minutes later and allow them to go home with the instruction to continue to drink more Naltrexone every 3 hours, but to stop and suck Buprenorphine if they get a significant withdrawal reaction.

If there is a withdrawal reaction then they still have opiates in their body. More Buprenorphineshould be sucked and Withdrawal Management Medications taken as needed. Further doses of Naltrexone should be withheld until the next day, depending on the strength of the reaction and the level of care available. This reaction means the patient is not yet clean enough to be on Naltrexone. The next day the process can begin again and be stopped and started until there is no reaction to larger doses and 2 litres of Naltrexone mixture (50mgm of naltrexone) has been consumed. The patient can then go onto 1 Naltrexone tablet every morning (or _ or _ or 1 _ or 2 tablets as needed and tolerated). There should be a compromise between taking the minimum dose that securely inhibits their craving for narcotics and the maximum dose that does not give them gut or nervous side effects. (nausea, anorexia, diarrhoea, anxiety/arousal, insomnia).

(ix) The popularity of naltrexone has waned considerably recently, due to side effects, cost, difficulties in achieving regularity of dosing and the worry as to whether there is an increased risk of O.D. in people who have been on naltrexone. If the patient doesn't want to go onto naltrexone, buprenorphine should be continued, perhaps at a reducing dose, until intense investigation and treatment of the Pre-existing Underlying Factors that caused and maintained the addiction, has reduced these Factors to the point where maintenance pharmacotherapy is not needed.

(x) Withdrawal of Methadone, which stays in the body for months and is highly addictive, has to be managed differently from withdrawal of other narcotics. If too much Buprenorphine is taken too quickly, a very uncomfortable Precipitated Withdrawal of the Methadone can occur. The best plan is to reduce the daily Methadone dose by 2 _ mgms. One mgm of Buprenorphine is then **sucked** when hanging out begins. 1mgm of Buprenorphine is repeated daily. After a few days the dose of Methadone is again reduced by 2 _ mgms. 1mgm of Buprenorphine continues to be sucked each day when hanging out begins. If the Buprenorphine makes the hanging out worse then a Precipitated Withdrawal is occurring. More Methadone should be given in extreme cases, although Clonidine and Clonazepam and reassurance will usually suffice in milder cases. If there is no sign of precipitated withdrawal then after a few days the Buprenorphine can be increased to 2mgms, then 4mgms daily and the Methadone reduced more rapidly. When the daily intake of Methadone has been reduced to 30mgms it can be stopped completely and 8mgms of Buprenorphine, or more as necessary, be sucked each day.

Buprenorphine can be continued, or Naltrexone can gradually be substituted six weeks after the last dose of Methadone. 40mls of a mixture of one 50mgm tablet crushed and well shaken in 2 litres of water (i.e. 1mgm of Naltrexone) is given every 7 days till it produces no reaction. The frequency of the dose can then be increased and when tolerated daily, the dose of Naltrexone is gradually increased. As the naltrexone is increasingly tolerated, the Buprenorphine can be slowly withdrawn.

Some treatment centers insist that patients get down to 30 to 40 mgm of Methadone before starting Buprenorphine. This means that those in greatest need are often not helped. It is extremely difficult, for most Methadone users on higher doses, to get down to 30 or 40 mgm of methadone. Many fail and drop out if they don't have small doses of Buprenorphine to help them reduce their Methadone to the "jumping off" level. However the Buprenorphine doses **must be small** and the Methadone addict can't, in the early stages, be given buprenorphine tablets to take home — they will nearly always take more than instructed and get into trouble with Precipitated Withdrawal, if given tablets to be taken home & selfadministered in the early stages.

(xi) In order to maintain the benefits of detoxification, **Maintenance Therapy and Underlying Factor Diagnosis and Correction** must be vigorously pursued. Some treatment centres just concentrate on switching people from street Narcotics and Methadone to ongoing Buprenorphine Maintenance Therapy. With Maintenance Therapy and Underlying Factor Correction, we get most of our patients completely clean of narcotics and most stay that way. About 10% are too unstable to maintain a clean state and need to be on longer term Maintenance Buprenorphine. In these cases it is particularly important to exclude ADD and Bipolar Disorder, perhaps with a trial of Dexamphetamine or Lithium, even if the patients don't appear to fit these diagnoses, as a common cause of failed detoxification is failure to recognize underlying ADD or Bipolar Disorder.

With Underlying Factor Diagnosis and Correction, ex addicts are less likely to need to stay on Buprenorphine, Naltrexone or other Maintenance Therapy Pharmaceuticals for long periods of time. The quality of their life is permanently improved and their vulnerability to Substance Abuse is reduced long term.

Unfortunately in Western Australia the rules with regard to prescribing and administering Buprenorphine have been changed so often in the last year or two, that there is doubt as to whether the authorities know what they are doing. Buprenorphine was first used for treating heroin addiction in Western Australia in the early 1980's, but then our Health Authorities stopped its use and promoted Methadone instead, from early 1984 onwards. They have been talking about doing trials to determine how Buprenorphine should be used, ever since. In my hands on experience of this extremely beneficial medicine I have not found it to be a difficult or dangerous chemical – certainly not nearly as dangerous as the street drugs or Methadone, which we are using it to displace. The shameful procrastination of the authorities has caused untold suffering and cost for addicts, their families and the community at large.

Current regulations mean that in W.A. we have difficulty administering Buprenorphine efficiently, according to an individual patient's needs and in such a way as to maximize the chances of successful detoxification. There are delays in getting the special permission needed to prescribe it, every dose has to be administered at a pharmacy & approval is not given to allow Methadone and Buprenorphine to the prescribed simultaneously for a patient. This precludes the gradual introduction of very small but increasing doses of buprenorphine, as the methadone is being gradually reduced, which is the surest and least traumatic way of getting methadone addicts off that terrible drug.

A person who needs 8mgms per day of Buprenorphine, but who vomits or has severe headaches if they take it all at once, under pharmacy supervision, as presently required, is not allowed to take part of the tablet under supervision and the rest at home, later in the day, which is how we did it before the second latest change of rules. The patient either has to suffer the headaches and vomiting, or to suffer withdrawals and perhaps failure in their detox attempt, by taking a smaller dose of Buprenorphine than they need.

One patient who was on 115mgm of Methadone daily and had never been able to reduce the dose before, is now down to 30mgm and progressing very well on 4mgms per day of Buprenorphine. He had to start on 1mgm per day of Buprenorphine and then gradually increase the dose, because to begin with, more than 1mgm at once caused a flare up of his asthma. The early doses also need to be kept to 1mgm or less, to avoid Precipitated Methadone Withdrawal in some people. Divided daily doses, are very difficult if all the doses have to be administered by a pharmacist at a pharmacy. The pharmacists naturally charge a fee for administering and doing the paper work for each dose, are usually not open 24 hours a day and the addicts don't have transport or money for multiple doses per day. There should be flexibility to allow the patient to take **small** quantities home, if several small doses are needed over the 24 hours, rather than taking just one larger dose per day at the clinic or pharmacy.

If a patient comes to the clinic hanging out, having already stopped his narcotics, it is essential that he be started on Buprenorphine immediately. If put off for a few days till a formal appointment can be made and permission to prescribe Buprenorphine is obtained – and this is what usually happens—the patient will usually get hold of illicit drugs, to relieve his acute withdrawal suffering, may commit crime to pay for them, and will often slip back to his old ways and contacts. It may then be months before he comes back again for detox and all sorts of bad things may happen in those months, to him, to his family and to other members of the community.

A few patients on Buprenorphine will want to go back to Methadone because on Methadone, when they can afford it or are offered it, they can have the pleasure of a shot of heroin, whereas with Buprenorphine, because of its blocking effect, heroin won't work.

NARCOTIC TOLERANCE AND DEATHS, FOLLOWING HEROIN TREATMENTS

One of the well known things about narcotics, is that when people take a narcotic, after repeated use they need more and more to produce the same effect. A person may start by getting relief or satisfaction from $25 worth of heroin, but soon need to take $100 or $200 worth per day. If they become a dealer or the partner of a dealer they may end up using and then needing $500 to $1000 worth per day. If for any reason their usage is stopped, within days or weeks their tolerance for heroin declines. This means that $25 worth will give them a result again and $200 worth may be enough to stop them breathing.

Therefore treating heroin addiction by any method, including cold turkey at home, in jail or in hospital, Rapid Detox or S.P.E.E.Q.E. Detox and Naltrexone, may be dangerous. Anyone who treats or manages heroin addicts must be extremely careful, as must ex addicts and their families and friends, or O.D. may be the end result. Detoxing is only safe if the Pre-existing, Underlying Causes of the addiction are diagnosed and treated successfully, or the patient is maintained on buprenorphine.

Addicts undergoing treatment must be clearly told over and over again that if they relapse, the first 4 hits after being clean must be no greater than the original dose which they used when they first started heroin. Also these initial 4 shots should be taken in the presence of unintoxicated people who can call an ambulance if breathing becomes shallow. The first four shots must also be taken when there has been no alcohol, benzodiazepines or other drugs consumed for many hours, as polydrug use often precedes O.D.

The Commonest Situations In Which There Is Danger Of Overdosing Are:

(1) Where the detoxed patient is still emotionally unstable due to undiagnosed or incompletely resolved Preexisting Underlying Factors that led to the original development of the addiction. The commonest of these factors are ADD, depression or manic depressive disorder, unresolved psychological and social traumas from the past, anxiety and panic disorder.

(2) Where sudden stresses occur, such as the breakdown of a relationship, the loss of access to a child, the death of a friend, motor vehicle accidents, arrest or court appearances and financial crises. At these times ex-addicts must be meticulous in making sure they don't miss one dose of their buprenorphine or naltrexone, or their craving will come back, they will use and be in danger of O.D. When they eventually stop their buprenorphine or naltrexone they should carry a few tablets with them at all times and take one at the first sign of temptation to use heroin. One buprenorphine or naltrexone tablet will give them 24 hours to get past the crisis, or if necessary, to resume buprenorphine or naltrexone maintenance therapy.

(3) When an ex-addict comes in contact with old acquaintances who are still using or dealing in drugs.

(4) Where alcohol, benzodiazepines or other drugs are affecting the addict at the time of the resumption of narcotic use.

A COMPREHENSIVE CHEMICAL HEALTH RECORD

For People who are excessive users of the social drugs caffeine, nicotine & alcohol or prescribed medications: for people who are dependent on, or addicted to, alcohol, cannabis, benzodiazapines, amphetamines, narcotics, cocaine, or other illegal drugs: for people who want to reassess themselves and any problems they suffer from, which may be giving rise to, or resulting from, their abnormal chemical intake: for people who want to make changes in their medications, social drug or hard drug usage.

Please download then complete as much as you can of this record, if necessary with the help of family, friends and healthcarers. Then take it to your usual family doctor or counsellor. If you wish, you can send your <u>completed</u> Comprehensive Chemical Health Record to Dr Beck for a written report on your condition and how it might possibly be managed. Please send with it one of the following fees (1) Standard Report $US40 (2) Comprehensive Report $US80 (3) Answers to Shorter Questions $US20 (4) Answers to More Detailed Questions $US30. Credit Card Details to www.CCNow.com. If you live in Western Australia you can make an appointment to see Dr Beck.

Family Name: _____

Forenames: _____ DOB: _____

Address: _____

_____ Postcode: _____

E-Mail: _____

Phone No's: _____

Medicare No: _____

Usual G.P or Healthcarer: _____

Date of First Consultation: _____

1. SUBSTANCES ABUSED & ADDICTIONS

Please **circle** any of the following chemicals that you have ever used. Put a second circle around the ones you have used in the last month **Cross out** the ones that you have never or almost never used. Put in the amounts or the **weekly** cost of the chemicals you are using now.

	First Consult	Reviews		
Dates				
Street Amphetamines age commenced				
Heroin age commenced				
Morphine or Other Narcotics age commenced				
Methadone				
Cannabis age commenced				
Valium, Serepax, Temazepam, or other Benzodiapines, (periods of more than 14 Benzodiapine tablets per week)				
Cocaine age commenced				
Rohypnol				
Caffeine (consistently more than 5 coffee or cola drinks per day)				
Nicotine (consistently more than 20 cigarettes per day) age commenced				
Alcohol (consistently more than 5 standard size alcoholic drinks per day) age commenced				
Petrol, Glue & Solvent Sniffing				
LSD				
Ecstasy age commenced				
Other Drugs				

Why do you think you started to use drugs in the first place?

What exactly is your desire & goal with regard to drugs?

Where do you rate your quality of life at present on a scale of 0-10 where 0 is horrible and 10 is perfect? 0 1 2 3 4 5 6 7 8 9 10 please circle the appropriate number.

Please **circle** any of the following things that apply to you, **cross out** the ones that don't apply to you, and **put a question mark** next to the ones that you are not sure about. Then, go back and put a second circle around the things that have affected you most.

2. FAMILIAL (INHERITED) DISORDERS

Have any of the members of your family or extended family, suffered from any of the following conditions? Anxiety, Panic Disorder, Sleep Disorders, Depression, Alcoholism, ADD, Bipolar Disorder, Schizophrenia, and other Mental illness. Have you been diagnosed with or do you think you might suffer from, any of these conditions?

_____

_____

_____

3. PHYSICAL DISEASE, INJURY AND CHRONIC PAIN

Head injury with loss of consciousness for more than 10 minutes, meningitis, epilepsy, chronic physical pain, other serious accidents injuries or illnesses

_____

_____

_____

4. EARLY CHILDHOOD FAMILY CIRCUMSTANCES

Death, Near Death, Serious Dysharmony or Separation of family members or parents from the family.

_____

_____

Verbal, Physical or Sexual Abuse of yourself, of any of your siblings or either of your parents (by whom?).

_____

_____

What were Your Main Sources of Love and Support in childhood? Were there any Family Members who should have been loving and supportive but weren't?

_____

_____

An unstable life, with Frequent Moves of Home, School (how many?) and Changes of Stepparents (how many?)

_____

_____

Immigration, War, Great Cultural or Socioeconomic Changes, Living In An Instituation.

_____

_____

5. ADOLESCENCE AND EARLY ADULT LIFE.

Difficulties with Education, Employment, Relationships, Housing, Money, Children, Frequent Moves, Rape or Abusive relationships, Disasters, Drug Users or Dealers close to you, Other Intolerable Circumstances. Problems in later life.

_____

_____

What have been the worst things in your life so far? What problems do you think about most? Is there or was there anything really bad that you have never told anybody about?

_____

_____

Do you have any Loves, Hopes, Dreams or Plans?

_____

_____

6. SIGNS OF CHEMICAL HEALTH and BRAINWAVE PROBLEMS

	First Consult	Reviews		
Dates				
Learning, Attention (Focus or Concentration) & Distractibility Problems, in the school years. At what level did you leave school?				
Inability to Stop Talking & Moving Around in school. Playing the Class Clown. Day Dreaming in class				
Impulsive Instantaneous Reactions, Decision Making & Actions or Procrastination & Inability to Make Decisions & to Get Started				
Do you seem to respond differently to amphetamines to the way most other people respond to amphetamines? Small doses of Dexamphetamine or Speed produce Calmness, No Rush, Improved Focusing, an Ability to Get Things Done, a sense of Feeling Normal?				
Great Impatience to get going at times, but at other times Hyperfocus and Getting Obsessed with things, with inability to move on to other necessary matters. Hurrying when there is no reason to hurry				
Periods of Too Much Energy and Activity or Periods of Abnormal Lack of Energy and Activity				

Intelligence, Talent or Giftedness in some things and complete inability in other things. Great variations in performance, depending on personal interest				
Depression. Suicidal Thoughts or Attempts				
Anxiety, Panic Attacks, Fear of Crowds, Phobias, Severe Agitation				
Inability to go to Sleep or to Stay Asleep				
Irritability, Temper, Rage, Aggression				
Flashbacks to Distressing Past Events				
Serious Highs with Hyperactivity, Talkativeness, Forcefulness, Grandiosity, Euphoria or Recklessness, sometimes alternating with Depression				
Paranoia, Hearing Voices, Thinking There are People in the Roof, Preoccupation with Extraterrestrial Things, Psychiatric Admissions				
Obsessiveness, Perfectionism, Repetitiveness, Workaholism, Sexaholism, Compulsive Gambling, Obsessive Compulsive Disorder				
Unusual Responses To Particular Medicines, Drugs, Drinks, Foods				
Poor response to, or inability to tolerate, some medications. (Please list them)				
Food Allergies, Unusual Cravings and Eating/Weight Disturbances, Anorexia, Bulemia				

For the doctor or psychologist to complete

PROBABLE PRE-EXISTING & UNDERLYING FACTORS LEADING TO SUBSTANCE ABUSE IN THIS CASE

The Main Past Addictions were
_____

The Main Present Addictions Are
_____

Please circle the factors suspected, then put a second circle around the most significant factors.

1. FAMILIAL (INHERITED) DISORDERS
_____

2. PHYSICAL DISEASE, INJURY OR CHRONIC PAIN
_____

3. EARLY CHILDHOOD TRAUMAS AND DEFICIENCIES
_____

4. ADOLESCENT AND EARLY ADULT LIFE TRAUMAS & DEFICIENCIES
_____

5. CHEMICAL HEALTH AND BRAINWAVE PROBLEMS

   (i).   **ADHD or ADDD (Very common)**
_____

   (ii).   **Anxiety, Stress, Depression (very common)**
_____

   (iii).   **Sleep Disorders (very common and usually secondary, but sometimes primary)**
_____

   (iv).   **Irritability, Temper, Rage, Aggression.**
_____

   (v).   **Post Traumatic Stress Disorders**
_____

   (vi).   **Bipolar (Manic Depressive) Disorder**
_____

   (vii).   **Psychosis, Drug Induced Psychosis**
_____

   (viii).   **Obsessive, Compulsive Disorder**
_____

6. OTHER PROBLEMS:

(i). **Personality Disorders**

(ii). **A "druggy" Family or Social Environment with many users, dealers, peer pressure or an addicted partner, family member or flatmate**

(iii). **Lack of Purpose in Life, Unemployment or lack of Responsibilities and Activities, Boredom, No Structure or Boundaries**

(iv). **Serious Sexual Problems including Abuse, Sexual Identity Conflict & the fear of "coming out"**

(v). **Other Factors or Health Disorders**

A MULTIDISCIPLINARY MANAGEMENT PLAN

1. **Serotonin Boosters** (SSRI's)
Efexor XR
Avanza
Cipramil

2. **Mood Stabilizers**
Sodium Valproate
Lithium
Clonazepam
Carbamazepine

3. **Agonists & Antagonists**
Buprenorphine
Naltrexone
Methadone

4. **"Stimulants"**
Dexamphetamine
Ritalin

5. **Tricyclics**
Doxepin
Amitryptiline

6. **Benzodiazapines**
Temazepam Tablets
Others

7. **Antipsychotics / Major Tranquillizers**
Zyprexa
Pericyazine

8. **Analgesics etc.**
Clonidine
Vioxx
Tramal SR
Panadeine Forte
Quinine Bisulphate
Buscopan
Losec / Somac
Tens Machine

9. **Other**

1. **Supply of Information**

   Information sheets on Buprenorphine, Detox Methods, ADD, Depression/anxiety, Diet, Groups, Medication, Meditation, EEG Biofeedback

   Books, Journals, Web Sites

   TV Programs & Videos, Edutainment Videos

2. **Shared Consultation Mini Marathons**

3. **One to One Counselling**

4. **Positive Group Therapy & Think Tanks**

5. **Psychiatric or Psychological Referral**

6. **EEG Biofeedback**

7. **Meditation**

8. **Further Education and Training**

9. **A New Home, Work, Partner, District, City or other Environmental Changes**

10. **Dietary Modification**

11. **Electromedicine**

12. **Acupuncture**

13. **Art Therapy**

14. **Music Therapy**

15. **Yoga**

16. **Communication, Relationship and Parenting Training**

17. **Other**

I have had this Multidisciplinary Management Plan explained to me and agree to work with it. I understand that anything I tell the doctor, nurse, psychologist or psychiatrist, is confidential but that they may discuss my confidential matters with one another, if it is thought that such discussion will further the understanding and treatment of my problems. I am happy to assist research into Chemical Health Problems and their causes and treatment, by allowing my Chemical Health Record to be studied by appropriate researchers, provided that in publishing their findings, my identity is not revealed and my privacy is fully respected.

Signed

PROGRESS NOTES

NAME : _____ **DOB:** _____

_____

_____

_____

_____

_____

_____

_____

_____

_____

_____

_____

_____

_____

_____

_____

_____

_____

_____

_____

_____

_____

_____

_____

_____

_____

_____

_____

_____

_____

A CURRENT MEDICATIONS RECORD

NAME: _____   DOB: _____

Medications Given	DATES:			
Serotonin Boosters				
Efexor XR				
Avanza				
Cipramil				
Mood Stabilisers				
Sodium Valproate				
Lithium				
Clonazepam				
Carbamazepine				
Buprenorphine				
Naltrexone				
Methadone				
"Stimulants"				
Dexamphetamine				
Ritalin				
Tricyclics				
Doxepin 25 mgm				
Amitryptiline 25mg				
Benzodiazapines				
Temazepam (Tablets)				
Diazepam				
Oxazepam				
Major Tranquillizers				
Zyprexa				
Pericyazine				
Analgesics				
Clonidine				
Vioxx 25 mgm				
Tramal SR				
Panadeine Forte				
Quinine Bisulphate				
Buscopan				
Losec / Somac				
Tens Machine				
The Patient's present Assessment of their **Quality Of Life** on a scale of 0 to 10				

A Psychosocial & E.E.G. Biofeedback Treatment Record

(Psychiatric reviews, psychologist, nurse-counsellor & EEG Biofeedback Sessions etc)

NAME: _____ **DOB:** _____

Date	Contact Type	Duration	Name Of Health Care Professional

A CASE REVIEW / RESULT ASSESSMENT/ NEW THREE MONTH MANAGEMENT PLAN

Name: DOB: Date First Seen:

Current Address:

Current Phone Nos:

Last 720 Review Date: Next Review No:

Date Due: Completion Confirmed

1. When they first came to this clinic, what exactly did this person think their main problems were?

_____

2. What exactly were they wanting to achieve?

   (a) Short Term

   (b) Longer Term

3. On a scale of 0 to 10 where did they rate their quality of life when first seen?   Now?

4. (a) What were their Substance Abuses when first seen?

   (b) What Other Substance Abuses had they previously had?

   Today's Date   (c) What Substance Abuses do they have now?

5. (a) What did we consider their main Preexisting Underlying Factors were during previous reviews?

   (i)

   _____

   (b) What Preexisting Underlying Factors do they have now?

   _____

6. Stage Of Treatment.   1. just started
2. on reduced drugs counselling established
3. midway
4. clean 3 months + adequate counselling
5. clean for 1 month + adequate counselling

7. Success So Far.   1. successful
2. unsuccessful
3. unsure (just started or relapse)

8. (a) What has worked well for them and what doesn't seem to work for them?

_____

(b) Pharmacotherapy recommended now

_____

(c) Other treatments recommended now

_____

(d) The Patient's Resolutions/ Goals for the next 3 months

_____

9. Other Comments

_____

10. Action to be taken, by whom and when?

_____

THE COMMONEST CAUSE OF SUBSTANCE ABUSE AND ADDICTION IS ADD

If ADD is the main cause of someone's addiction, but the ADD is not discovered and treated, the health care professionals involved might almost as well not start to treat the addiction. The addiction will keep recurring again and again. If the addiction is to heroin, overdosing will be a danger during these repeated treatments. Each time the addict gets off the heroin, which has been controlling the ADD suffering, that suffering will flare up again, causing the addict to again seek relief through cannabis, street amphetamines and then heroin.

What is Attention Deficit Disorder? It is a chemical disorder of the brain. We have approximately 140 different chemicals in our brain and it is believed that ADD is caused by inheriting faulty genes, which result in faulty regulation of the supply of four of the most important brain chemicals. They are Dopamine, Adrenalin, Noradrenaline and Serotonin. ADD is also an electrical disorder of the brain. The electrical waves of the brain, as measured by an EEG, are different in patients with ADD. They indicate disturbances in a fundamental feature of brain function – the level of arousal.

These abnormalities give rise to a vicious cycle of poor functioning, discomfort and distress and the use of drugs to try to boost performance and relieve distress. Those drugs usually cause more problems than they solve, thus putting the ADD sufferer into ever increasing distress and trouble.

Although the different aspects of ADD vary in degree from person to person, the common pattern is as follows.

There is poor attention, focusing or concentration. This leads to learning difficulties and a poor education.

There is a disturbance of activity, usually overactivity and hurrying (Attention Deficit Hyperactivity Disorder, or Attention Deficit Hurry Disorder, or ADHD); but sometimes resulting in underactivity, boredom, daydreaming, slowness, dawdling and lack of motivation, with difficulty in getting started and a tendency to procrastinate (Attention Deficit Daydreaming Disorder or ADDD). This activity disorder may result in problems in the classroom. The child cannot stop talking, fidgeting or moving around, distracting his classmates, aggravating his teachers and perhaps becoming the class clown; or he/she may sit quietly in the corner of the class daydreaming, be neglected and fall behind. The family may be driven mad, and relationships be strained or damaged, because of the hyperactivity and impatience, or because of failure to achieve and to contribute. Employment is very difficult, with poor performance, friction with employers and workmates and frequent dismissals, resignations and periods of unemployment.

There is a strong tendency to impulsivity, with knee jerk reactions and snap decisions the norm, often resulting in mistakes, regrets & overuse of credit cards or shoplifting.

There are often problems with time. ADD people are often very impatient and 5 minutes may seem or be an impossible length of time for them to wait. On the other hand they may get so involved in things that they don't notice the hours going by, miss meals, neglect other duties and forget appointments. Appointments are very hard for ADD sufferers to make and to keep. They often can't come to grips with making an appointment with a psychiatrist who has a six week waiting list. They often have difficulty with things that require planning ahead.

The net result of all this is that education and performance is poor, relationships are strained, there may be difficulty in getting or keeping a job and certainly in developing a satisfactory career, and the suffering and distress involved may mean that the person seeks relief through various types of social, prescribed or illegal drugs. This tendency to substance abuse is so common that ADD sufferers are sometimes said to have an "addictive brain". Any person who has a history of significant use of amphetamines, cannabis and narcotics, past or present, almost certainly suffers from ADD. Research recently showed that treatment of primary school ADD children with Dexamphetamine or Ritalin, reduces their chances of substance abuse in adolescence by 85%.

It is our finding, confirmed by independent psychiatric assessment in most cases, that at least 60% of the heroin addicts I see in my clinic are ADD sufferers, mostly ADHD sufferers, but also a significant number of ADDD sufferers.

The Treatment Of ADD Consists Of:

1. Reducing the chemical abnormalities by the use of Dexamphetamine or Ritalin, which have a normalising effect rather than a stimulating effect on ADD sufferers. Dexamphetamine and Ritalin are difficult to obtain because both the public and the authorities have tended to lump them together with other dangerous black market amphetamines such as Speed and Methamphetamine and to overlook the fact that ADD sufferers have unusual chemistry. One man's poison is literally another man's medicine with ADD. In most developed countries the baby has been thrown out with the bath water. Much damage is being done to innocent people by regulations which were introduced to protect the population against addiction, but which are based on faulty generalisations that cause a very vulnerable section of the population, who don't have the resources or the capabilities to get proper medical attention and pharmaceuticals, to use dangerous and unsatisfactory alternatives from drug dealers.

2. E.E.G. Biofeedback if available and affordable.

3. Any other concurrent substance abuse must be effectively diagnosed and treated.

4. Any other disturbances such as depression, anxiety, social phobia or relationship or family breakdowns, that coexist with or have been brought on by the ADD, must be dealt with.

5. Assessments should be done to·define the gaps in the sufferer's education, caused by their inattention and inability to focus/concentrate and their behaviour problems and strained classroom relationships, during their school years. Supplementary education should be used to fill in the gaps and complete their education.

6. Training will be needed to make use of their new ability to focus/concentrate, read and study and their normalized energy/activity, in preparing for employment and a career.

7. If legal Dexamphetamine or Ritalin is not available (which is the scandalous situation that exists in Perth for any adult who cannot afford to consult a private psychiatrist) then Epilim (Sodium Valproate), serotonin boosters and tricyclics will usually have some beneficial effect. The alternative is black market Dexamphetamine or Ritalin, taken in the morning by mouth, regularly and in small amounts. Black market Dexamphetamine or Ritalin is a far safer and better choice than intravenous street amphetamines, heroin or cocaine, if a sufferer has to make do with self medication for a period.

In Western Australia the only free public clinic that diagnoses and treats ADD is the children's hospital. Family doctors, even if they are experts in drug and alcohol medicine, cannot prescribe stimulant therapy. This means that penniless addicts have to go without proper treatment and usually self medicate dangerously, using cannabis, intravenous street amphetamines, heroin, morphine, or cocaine, at a cost that causes poverty and crime and brings the risks of Hepatitis B and C and HIV.

Because of some of the genes many of us carry, a proportion of our babies are born with genes that inevitably lead to unusual chemistry, which almost inevitably leads to conditions (ADD, depression, anxiety etc) that in turn almost inevitably lead to distress, poor performance, social problems, substance abuse and dependence and great social cost. Fortunately today we have the capability to correctly diagnose & treat those conditions, although unfortunately it often doesn't happen.

Until the healthcare professionals, the public generally and the authorities in this field, understand and act on ADD, this whole sequence will continue to occur and drug addiction, the drug world and the drug lords will grow and prosper.

We must provide reasonable availability of chemicals that relieve these chemically unusual and afflicted people of their distress and disability, without giving rise to the side effects and dangers of the drugs and methods pushed by the criminal world.

We already have the chemicals we need – buprenorphine, valproate, serotonin boosters, naltrexone, dexamphetamine, ritalin, and occasionally lithium, but so far we lack the wisdom and systems to make them reasonably available. Available in ways that are accessible even to people who suffer from the disabilities, dysfunctions and lack of resources of ADD sufferers.

Despite anything anyone may tell you, none of these types of medicine is any more dangerous than dozens of other chemicals your family doctor writes prescriptions for every week. If they were reasonably available, in a way that was accessible to people with the disabilities and dysfunctions ADD sufferers have, there would be very little street trade in any of them. The criminal market for speed, methamphetamine, ecstasy, heroin, morphine, cocaine and cannabis would contract sharply. The pushers and the Mr. Bigs would have to find something else to do. The Criminal Justice, Education and Public Hospital systems would have the pressure taken off them. We would be able to get on with building up the people we are presently causing untold misery and chopping to pieces.

S.N. age 38, male

When I first attended Dr Beck's clinic I was on a disability pension, unemployable and on antidepressant and antipsychotic medications from a government psychiatric clinic. I was being kept poor by the cost of intravenous speed, which I couldn't do without. Previously I had used LSD, marijuana and alcohol for my emotional disturbances.

My desire was to stop using amphetamines, to not always be broke, to control my temper, to get into the workforce and to have a normal life. I had tried to get off amphetamines about once a year, but usually only succeeded for a week.

Other things that I suffered from were sleeplessness, depression, anxiety and panic attacks, perfectionism, social phobia, severe agitation, violent outbursts, compulsive gambling and sexuality, suicidal thoughts and alcoholism. I was physically abused by my father and had been in jail for a year because of my violence. I lost my brothers because of my aggression and violence.

I did badly at school and could never concentrate. The only employment I ever got was labouring. The longest relationship I had managed only lasted a month. I lived on my own.

I wanted to be settled, to stop being violent, to be able to concentrate, to have better relationships and more motivation, to stop using drugs and to not always be financially out of control.

At the first consultation Dr Beck completed an ADD questionnaire on me and told me that my problem was severe ADD. He gave me twelve dexamphetamine tablets to try over a two day period. It totally changed me. I felt much calmer, was able to concentrate, was more motivated and much more able to get things done and I didn't feel aggressive or violent. He also put me on Epilim, 500 mg in the morning and 1000 mg in the evening, which he said sometimes helps with ADD when dexamphetamine is not available.

Dr Beck then referred me to a psychiatrist because only a psychiatrist could prescribe dexamphetamine for me on an ongoing basis in Western Australia. The psychiatrist interviewed both me and my girlfriend and agreed with the diagnosis of ADD. He put me on daily dexamphetamine and my life has been transformed. I was able to stop the antipsychotic medication, the antidepressants and the intravenous amphetamines. I felt clear, relaxed, not bored, not fidgety and my aggression and temper resolved completely. I also have been able to stop the cannabis quite easily. I soon had some money in my pocket. I have now found a part time job as a kitchen hand, with good prospects that this work will become full time. Dr Beck tells me I am intelligent. My aim now is to go to university to get a decent education and a qualification and Dr Beck says he is confident that I will be able to achieve this.

I tried stopping my dexamphetamine for one day, but all my symptoms came back. I went back on the dexis again and I now feel normal and settled and have been consistently happy for the first time in my life, that I can remember. My dexis were stolen once when I let an old addict friend stay overnight because he had nowhere else to go. Until I could get more dexis I kept on having accidents & breaking plates. My employers were unhappy with me because of this & I had to explain what was going on. When I got more dexis I was better again & they were happy with me again & increased my hours and pay.

AN ADD DIAGNOSTIC QUESTIONNAIRE & TREATMENT RECORD FOR ADOLESCENTS & ADULTS

(ADD = Attention Deficit Disorder = Focusing/Activity/Impulsivity/Time/ Disorder & Suffering)

1. How Did You Get On In Primary School?

(a) Did you have difficulties with learning? If so, what were some of the difficulties that you had? **(YES/NO)**

(b) Did you have behaviour which was disturbing to your teachers or to your classes (e.g. excessive talking or movement). How did your teachers react to this behaviour? What did they do to you? **(Y/N)**

2. How Did You Get On In High School?

(a) Did you have learning difficulties? If so, what learning difficulties? Were there some subjects you were good at and others you were bad at? If so, which subjects? **(Y/N)**

(b) Did you have behaviour which upset your teachers or disturbed your classes? If so, what were the problems? How did your teachers react to this behaviour? What did they do to you? **(Y/N)**

(c) Were you away from school a lot? For what reasons? What did you do on the days you didn't go to school? **(Y/N)**

(d) How many Primary Schools did you attend? Which High Schools did you attend?

(e) In what year of school did you leave? During term or at the end of the term or the year? Why did you leave?

3. At what time do you prefer to go to bed and at what time do you prefer to get up? Do you have difficulty going to sleep or getting up? Please give details.

_____

_____

4. Do you sometimes find it hard to get motivated, to get started? Do you often procrastinate and get behind in things? Do you often daydream? (Y/N)

_____

_____

5. Are you a very active person? Do you tend to have several things on the go at once? Do you start new things before you finish what you are already doing? Do you have difficulty finishing things? (Y/N)

_____

_____

6. If you get interested or involved in something, or focused on something, do you tend to get so wrapped up in it that you don't notice the time going by and neglect other things? (Y/N)

_____

_____

7. Are you often in a hurry? Do you often get very restless, impatient, unable to wait, or to wait your turn? (Y/N)

_____

_____

8. Do you often make decisions & act or react very quickly? Do you often regret these quick decisions? (Y/N)

_____

_____

9. Have you had problems in your employment? If so, what problems? (Y/N)

_____

_____

10. Have you had problems in your relationships? If so, what problems? (Y/N)

_____

_____

11. What types of unhappiness and distress, if any, do you experience?

_____

_____

12. Do you, or have you in the past, abused any drugs or substances? If so, what were they and how much was your maximum usual daily amount. (Y/N)

_____

_____

13. If you use a small amount (1 to 3 points) of amphetamine, what effect does it have on you?

_____

If you use a larger amount (half to one gram) what effect does it have on you?

_____

14. Are there any foods, confectionary, drinks or other substances that seem to make you (or anyone else in your family) sleepless, restless, overactive, irritable or aggressive? Are you allergic to gluten or dairy products? Do you eat a lot of junk food, sugar or confectionary, or drink a lot of cordials or canned or bottled drinks? (Y/N)

_____

_____

15. Have you ever been charged or fined for any offences? If so, what offences and what were the outcomes? (Y/N)

_____

_____

16. Have you ever seen a psychologist, a psychiatrist or any other doctor or counsellor about any psychological or social problems? If so, what was their diagnosis of your problems? What treatments did they recommend or give to you? What were their names? (Y/N)

_____

_____

17. Circle any of the following that you or members of your extended family have, or have suffered.

a)   High IQ, originality or inventiveness (Y/N)

_____

b)   Sporting, artistic, musical or literary talent (Y/N)

---

c)   Head injuries, brain disease or epilepsy (Y/N)

---

d)   Severe pain or sleeplessness (Y/N)

---

e)   Depression, manic depressive disorder or post traumatic stress (Y/N)

---

f)   Anxiety, panic attacks, phobias, social phobia or severe agitation (Y/N)

---

g)   Obsessive compulsive disorder or perfectionism (Y/N)

---

h)   Violent outbursts, rage, serious anti-social behaviour (Y/N)

---

i)   ADD, ADHD or ADDD, workaholism, compulsive gambling, spending or sexuality (Y/N)

---

j)   Hearing Voices, paranoia, schizophrenia or other psychosis, psychiatric hospital admissions or any other mental illness or sexual deviance (Y/N)

---

k)   Suicidal thoughts or attempts or unexplained deaths (Y/N)

---

l)   Emigration, family breakdown or deaths, financial, jail, war or other horrible experiences (Y/N)

---

m) Anorexia, bulimia, allergy or sensitivity to any foods, drinks or confectionary, etc (Y/N)

---

n)   Heavy consumption of alcohol, caffeine, nicotine or cannabis (Y/N)

FOR THE HEALTHCARE PROFESSIONAL TO COMPLETE
Differential Diagnosis and Comorbidities

(a) **Misbehaviour due to High IQ, Giftedness and Boredom: (Y/N)**

_____

(b) **Deep Seated Anxiety: (Y/N)**

_____

(c) **Manic Depressive Disorder: (Y/N)**

_____

(d) **Other Comorbidities e.g. Dissociative or Personality Disorder, Tics, Dyskinesia, Tourette's: (Y/N)**

_____

(e) **Schizophrenia, Psychosis, an over stimulated state that may be aggravated by Stimulant Therapy: (Y/N)**

_____

(f) **Undiagnosed Drug, Alcohol or Benzodiazepine Abuse: (Y/N)**

_____

(g) **ADD, ADHD or ADDD**   **(i) Mild:** _____

   (ii) Moderate: _____

   (iii) Severe: _____

(h) **Other:**

_____

_____

A MULTIDISCIPLINARY MANAGEMENT PLAN

ADD is a difficult and very significant problem, capable of ruining a person's life, as well as the life of their family. If you suspect from the above questionnaire that you might have it, you need to be assessed by a psychiatrist <u>who specialises in this field</u>, to confirm the diagnosis of ADD, as well as the diagnosis of any other conditions that may coexist. The proper treatment of ADD includes education, therapy and medication – you need all three. A psychiatrist is the best place to start, because they have the knowledge to confirm the diagnosis and to get you started on all three types of treatment. You will then probably be directed on to a psychologist or classes or groups.

(a) Immediate Relief & Medications:

_____

(b) Recommended Specialists, Psychotherapy & Counselling, EEG Biofeedack:

_____

(c) Recommended Education & Career Development:

_____

(d) Patient Declaration: I have had this management plan explained to me and discussed with me. I am in agreement with it and will follow it through. I am happy to contribute to the knowledge of and treatment for ADD sufferers by hereby giving permission to my doctor to allow appropriate research workers to study this record, provided my identity is not made public in any way.

Signed: _____ Date: _____

(e) If You Can't Get Proper Treatment:

For various reasons, some people cannot get proper treatment for ADD and continue to self medicate with street amphetamines and/ or cannabis and/ or narcotics, or to be treated by people who cannot prescribe Ritalin or Dexamphetamine. If you can't get full professional help and prescribing and are treating yourself with illicit drugs and getting some benefit, you will get much more benefit if you;

(i)   take epilim (valproate) 500mgms 1 tablet in the morning and 1 or 2 tablets in the evening

(ii) try to find a street source of Dexamphetamine or Ritalin tablets and take them orally with the same dose each breakfast and lunchtime, once you find the best dose, by trial and error, rather than using street speed intravenously or

(iii) take small doses of speed every morning rather than large doses irregularly every few days.

AN UNPUBLISHED "LETTER TO THE EDITOR"

Albany Highway Chemical Health Centre

DR NEIL BECK
Provider No: 187242H
A.B.N. No: 66 900 952 705

12 April 2001
The Editor
The Washington Post

Dear Sir/Madam,

With regard to your article of the 18/3/01 **The Trouble With ADHD**.

Researchers put the number of different chemicals in the human brain, at between one and two hundred. This large number of different chemicals is the basis of our diverse and sophisticated brain function. Given the variety of genetic, nutritional, toxic, disease related and traumatic factors that may effect any particular person's brain, from the embryonic stage onwards, we should not expect all people's brain chemicals and functioning to be the same. There may be an excess, a deficiency or an imbalance, of any of the numerous brain chemicals and brain chemical systems.

These excesses, deficiencies and imbalances may cause excessive, reduced, or unusual responses to other chemicals which reach the brain from foods, drinks, medicines or drugs. This in turn may add to the variations in brain function, affecting thinking, feeling and behaviour. Working in the field of drug and alcohol medicine, I have found that it is very helpful to operate on the basis that 80 to 90% of the population have "usual" brain chemistry and 10 to 20% have "unusual" brain chemistry. Amongst addicts the percentage who have "unusual" brain chemistry is very much higher, so that when you prescribe treatment for them, you have to be prepared for outcomes which may be quite different from what you expected.

ADD is the commonest and one of the most disastrous forms of "unusual" chemistry. It is due to a number of faulty genes that can give rise to unusual/abnormal regulation of the supply of the brain chemicals dopamine, adrenaline, noradrenaline and serotonin.

As a result of their particular "unusual" chemistry, ADD sufferers either have difficulty in paying attention, or attend too intensely; are overactive and excessively impulsive, or can't get started and tend to daydream and procrastinate; can't wait a minute or just don't notice many hours going by; and are often very vulnerable to drugs, especially cannabis, amphetamines and heroin, which give them some relief from their "unusual chemistry" induced malfunctioning and distress. Any person who has used any or all of these three drugs, needs to be assessed for ADD.

A combined chemical, psychosocial, educational and dietary approach is highly desirable, to achieve maximum success in managing ADD. One of these approaches on it's own will not give as good or as quick a result as a combined approach.

Unfortunately the diversity of knowledge needed for this combined approach is too much for one person to cover; but once different professions are covering different parts of the problem, you start to get conflicts. I am very pro counselling, therapy, education and diet, but would like to provide some additional information, based on personal experience, to support a chemical element to the approach to managing ADD.

There are four medicines which I have found useful in treating ADD. Epilim (sodium valproate) is completely safe (and therefore easy to get), gives considerable immediate relief to overactive and agitated ADHD sufferers and is valuable first aid, especially for people who are in acute trouble with drugs. Venlafaxine (Efexor XR) and Doxepin are safe, easy to get and well worth a try, especially for those ADD patients who are also depressed. Dexamphetamine and Ritalin are usually much more effective than Epilim or Venlafaxine, but are controversial and generally difficult to obtain. I find them to be quite safe if handled wisely, but they are often not handled wisely.

There are at least four factors that make Dexamphetamine and Ritalin controversial and difficult to obtain, to the detriment of individuals and families who are affected by ADD.

Firstly ADD sufferers have "unusual" chemistry and respond differently to Dexamphetamine and Ritalin than do people with "usual" chemistry. If you ask people who don't have ADD how they respond to amphetamines they will tell you they get a rush or a high and can't relax or sleep. If you ask ADD sufferers what amphetamines do to them, they will say they become more relaxed, focused and "normal," can get things done that they should have done a long time ago and can go to sleep, unless they take large doses. (Asking this question is a good way of helping to diagnose ADD).

The statement that is sometimes made that "it is silly to give stimulants to hyperactive children" sounds very sensible, but is based on the flawed concept that everyone has the same brain chemistry and responds to medications in the same way. They don't. Ritalin and Dexamphetamine are **not** stimulants but are in a sense sedatives for ADD sufferers. ADD sufferers have "unusual" chemistry and respond to these medicines in the opposite way to non-ADD people. Nevertheless the apparent common sense of not giving stimulants to hyperactive people, has made it more difficult for ADD sufferers to obtain this highly effective treatment.

Secondly, unfortunately the baby has been thrown out with the bathwater in regard to Ritalin and Dexamphetamine. ADD, with the inner distress it causes, the damage to the ability to learn, the compromised education and therefore compromised career and finances of the sufferer, the illicit drug problems and the damage to relationships, causes ADD sufferers to make up a substantial proportion of the most distressed, poor, degraded, criminal and costly members in most communities. Yet the diagnosis of ADD is usually not very difficult to make and the chemical aspect of the treatment is easy, dramatically effective and comparatively inexpensive, safe, effective and easy to supervise. So why let so much ADD continue untreated, with all its life wrecking and community disrupting consequences?

Once again problems have been caused by flawed generalisations. Many parents, healthcarers and authorities have, in their mind, lumped Ritalin and Dexamphetamine together with street amphetamines. Dexamphetamine and Ritalin are medicines, synthesized in proper registered pharmaceutical laboratories, by reputable registered internationally known pharmaceutical companies and dispensed by qualified registered pharmacists to ADD sufferers through prescriptions written by highly qualified, specialist doctors. Speed or street amphetamines are a hotch potch of multiple raw materials, based on varying recipes, manufactured by unscrupulous criminals, with whatever chemicals they have on hand at the time, in backyard kitchens with uncertain precision and cleanliness and sold by other unscrupulous criminals, often in unhygienic circumstances, to anyone who will pay. "Stimulant" therapy for ADHD is a totally different thing to the black market in street amphetamines and yet many people, in ignorance and fear, lump them together and condemn Dexamphetamine and Ritalin because of a false perception that all amphetamines are much of a muchness. This means that many ADD sufferers don't get treated and resort to erratically self administered unsafe street amphetamines.

The third problem is that the legal distribution of Ritalin and Dexamphetamine for the treatment of ADD is carried out in general in the same way that we distribute other medications – and it shouldn't be. Doctors are used to giving patients on long-term therapy, prescriptions for a month's supply or for 100 or 200 tablets at a time. Although Dexamphetamine is a pretty tame chemical compared to the speedy cocktails crims cook up, it still can be sold and kids and addicts enjoy the intrigue and the profits of dealing in it. The prescriptions must therefore specify that the pharmacist should dispense only 2 to 7 day's supply at a time. Some pharmacists will complain about the extra work but genuine, professional pharmacists will understand the reasons for doing this and readily comply. The patients then do not get enough tablets at one time to make a sale that would be sufficient to pay for a hit of heroin. They cannot use their month's dexamphetamine all in the first week and then suffer from active ADD for the next three weeks. They can't lose or have stolen, 3 or 4 weeks' supply in one hit, as ADD people so often seem to do, and then be in great distress till the next supply becomes available.

The fourth problem is that Dexamphetamine and Ritalin can only be prescribed by Pediatricians, Neurologists and Psychiatrists in many countries. However for ADD sufferers, who are often penniless and too disturbed to make and keep appointments, and who may even have difficulty in sitting in a doctor's waiting room for 10 minutes, this creates an impossible situation. For this reason a great proportion of the black market in street amphetamines is carried out by self-medicating ADD sufferers, for whom the correct channels are almost impossible. The rules and regulations that are meant to protect sick people, actually force severe adult ADD sufferers to mix in the criminal world, to use defective treatments, and alienate them from healthcare professionals, who could arrange the psychological, social, educational and dietary advice which they need, in addition to the chemicals, in order to recover from the effects of their ADD.

ADD is, in my experience, the commonest cause of severe cannabis abuse and of narcotic and amphetamine addiction. This group of addicts is the easiest to diagnose and treat. Correct pharmacotherapy immediately results in enormous benefit to them, their families and their communities. Why aren't we getting on and diagnosing and treating them?

Yours sincerely,

Neil Beck.

I.S. female, age 43.

At my first Shared Consultation with Dr Beck I was covered in bruises, as usual, from fist fighting with my flatmate. I was also, as usual, very tense and agitated and kept moving from one chair to another. I hadn't slept for 5 days. Dr Beck usually works with groups of patients all together and I found what the other patients said, and what Dr Beck asked them and told them, very interesting. I asked Dr Beck and the other patients some questions, but I couldn't tell my story in front of the group, so Dr Beck then took me into a private consulting room by myself.

I told him I had been a problem from birth and that I had been diagnosed as having ADHD when I was a little girl. My parents were poor and couldn't keep up with the cost of the dexamphetamine which was prescribed for me, so it was stopped even though it helped me. I told Dr Beck I had been in jail many times, once for six years. He put me on four doxepin 25 mgm tablets at 7.00pm each evening and told me to try to get a few black market dexamphetamines as he couldn't prescribe these himself and it would take many weeks and be very expensive to see a psychiatrist about this problem. He then told me to come back in 2 days.

I managed to get some dexis and was absolutely amazed at the results as I had the two best nights sleep I could remember for years and had two days in which I was not violent. It made me very sad and angry to think of all I had been through, and all the trouble I had caused, because I wasn't able to have the medicine I needed.

I went on taking 8 dexis and feeling good on the days when I could get them, but sometimes used up to $200 worth of I.V. speed when I couldn't get the dexis. Sometimes I couldn't sleep and when I couldn't sleep I would eat non-stop and do obsessive house cleaning. Dr Beck then tried Zyprexa, a major tranquilizer, with some benefit. I am now waiting for assessment by a psychiatrist.

I am much better than I was and feel hopeful for the first time in my life, of getting to the bottom of my problems and understanding and managing them. I just wish it was quicker and easier for ADD sufferers to get diagnosed and treated. It would save a great deal of pain and suffering for everybody and stop the drug dealers getting fat while sick people go through hell

DEPRESSION/ ANXIETY/ STRESS & INSOMNIA

Our clinical impression and the analysis of 121 consecutive cases indicates that ADD is the commonest <u>cause</u> of substance abuse and addiction, amongst patients attending the Albany Highway Chemical Health Centre. However the commonest clinical conditions found amongst our patients are those of depression/ anxiety/ stress and insomnia; sometimes as the <u>cause</u> and sometimes as the <u>effect</u> of the addiction. ADD leads to substance abuse and addiction, but addiction does not lead to ADD. However depression/ anxiety/ stress and insomnia, may be a partial or the sole cause of an addiction, or addiction may result in depression/ anxiety/ stress/ insomnia. In fact these clinical conditions are present in almost all of our patients and how well we manage them is a very important factor in whether we succeed or fail in treating the addiction.

Amongst our most severe and difficult cases of addiction there are some people who have been profoundly depressed for many years, sometimes from early childhood. Some of the most difficult cases also suffer from both depression and ADD. 10% suffer from Manic Depressive (Bipolar) Disorder, with or without comorbid ADD. These are the addiction cases most likely to be incompletely diagnosed and where treatment is most likely to be inadequate and therefore unsuccessful. If an addiction patient is not getting better, these are the conditions to look for. These are conditions which, when mixed with substance abuse and missed diagnoses, can totally ruin a person's life and the life of their family.

Depression is very common and significant amongst addicts – about 71% in our review. One of the major problems we often come across, is depressed people, suffering from substance abuse or addiction, who refuse to take antidepressants. They say they have been put on various antidepressants in the past, but that the antidepressants didn't help them. What I have found is that when you are treating a general population of depressed patients, even if the first antidepressant doesn't work, the second or third one probably will. However when you are treating an addict population, both you and they have to be prepared to go through anything up to six or more antidepressants, before you find one which lifts the burden of depression. Usually, until you find an antidepressant regime that works for them, it is very difficult for these patients to stay off illicit drugs, and they will continually harass you for more and more benzodiazapines.

Another interesting thing that we have found is that if we treat addicted depression patients with up to 100mg of a Tricyclic Antidepressant, such as doxepin or amitryptiline, at 7pm each evening, together with a Serotonin Booster such as Avanza, Efexor XR or Cipramil, then almost invariably the depression will lift quite satisfactorily. This will then greatly change and improve the patient's life and their attitude to and response to treatment. This process, known as Augmentation, can also be carried out using Lithium or Zyprexa in conjunction with Serotonin Boosters. The augmentation medication chosen initially, a Tricyclic, Lithium or Zyprexa, should depend on any comorbid conditions or other tendencies the patient suffers from. A tricyclic is usually the best where anxiety and insomnia are a big problem in addition to the depression; lithium where there is a tendency to manic behaviour; Zyprexa where there is a tendency to psychosis.

This raises the question of overdose deaths in the addict population. My approach to that risk has eventually become to invariably only prescribe the 25mg strength of Doxepin or Amitryptiline and to specify on the prescription that the pharmacist should only dispense twenty-five of these tablets at one time and not more often than once in every six days. I have found that the reduction in risk behaviour that this treatment gives, far outweighs any increase in risk it may create. I have never had a death occur in any of my drug and alcohol patients.

Anxiety/ panic attacks/ panic disorder/ stress and insomnia are very often described by patients. They are the common curse of substance abusers, whether they are the cause of their abuse or the result of their roller coaster addict life. They are a very important aspect of the assessment/ diagnosis and treatment of addiction patients. It is very difficult to beat drugs until the anxiety/ stress and insomnia are under control. The interesting thing is that by a process of learning from our problems with really difficult patients, we eventually came to the conclusion that the treatment for anxiety/stress and insomnia, is very similar to the most effective treatment for depression; and that all of these problems are often best treated in the same way and as the one condition. The EEG Biofeedback (Neurofeedback) practitioners would probably tell us not to be surprised at this finding. They would probably tell us that all these conditions have the same origin – an underlying disturbance of arousal in the brain

Early in my work with drug and alcohol patients, I worked with some doctors who were very free in their prescribing of benzodiazapines (benzos). Many people were supplied quite freely with flunitrazepam (Rohypnol or rohies), nitrazepam (Mogadon), diazepam (Valium), and oxazepam (Serepax) as well as the usual temazepam. It was common to find patients who were taking twenty-five benzodiazepines per day. I met one small female who was taking six to eight flunitrazepam and eight to ten nitrazepam in 24 hours and still had the greatest of difficulty in sleeping. She also suffered from serious anxiety and depression. I met one patient who was taking a hundred benzodiazapines per day and still couldn't sleep (he had undiagnosed Bipolar Disorder). Benzodiazapine dependence or addiction was the fourth-commonest dependence in our study of 121 consecutive patients at the Albany Highway Chemical Health Centre. Approximately 38% of our patients suffer from this form of substance abuse, usually in conjunction with other substance abuses. This type of medication seemed to me to be a failure and to cause more problems than it solved. With considerable patient resistance, I have moved against it since establishing my own my clinic. My experience is that when the going gets tough for an addict, benzos in ever increasing amounts won't resolve the anxiety, won't give a good sleep and often make depression worse.

The medications which in the end proved to be the best solution for anxiety/stress and insomnia, were the ones which we had already found to be the best solution for depression. We now basically prescribe 50-100mg of Tricyclic antidepressant at 7pm, usually with one Serotonin Booster SSRI tablet per day. We will prescribe temazepam tablets (not capsules) at bedtime because of temazepam's short half-life and its effectiveness in putting people to sleep (even though it doesn't keep them asleep, a problem which we usually overcome with doxepin). We have cut out temazepam capsules because of the severity of the physical (e.g. amputations) and psychological problems caused if they are injected intravenously (as one patient put it, I.V. temazepam gives a Rohypnol type effect). We are very reluctant to prescribe diazepam or oxazepam and only prescribe them in very limited quantities in special situations, and to be dispensed only a few days supply at a time by the pharmacy. We never ever prescribe flunitrazepam and rarely prescribe nitrazepam and then only as a temporary compromise deal with a new patient. We find that there is a small role for clonazepam as a mood stabilizer, but we watch it very carefully as people often rapidly become dependant on it. Otherwise Tricyclic and SSRI Antidepressants (Serotonin Boosters), with the occasional addition of pericyazine or olanzapine (Zyprexa), are used instead of benzodiazepines, for anxiety/ stress and insomnia, as well as for depression.

It is very important to realise that ADD is often misdiagnosed as anxiety/ insomnia and that these symptoms are then often treated with the wrong medicines, which make the condition worse. ADHD certainly may appear and feel like anxiety. Insomnia or sleep disturbances certainly are a large part of ADHD. Which the problem is may become apparent by careful questioning of the patient about their reactions to amphetamines and benzos. Amphetamines in small doses will make the ADD patient calmer, more focused, more "normal" ("I feel more normal doc") and more able to sleep, while benzos make little difference or may make them worse. Benzos will make the anxiety patient better temporarily, whilst amphetamines will make them worse.

DIET IS SIGNIFICANT IN TREATING HEROIN ADDICTION

If substance abuse proneness and addiction in our communities, are partly due to some members of these communities having disturbed or unusual chemistry, then it seems likely that the chemicals these people daily feed into themselves, in what they eat and drink, could be a factor in their substance abuse and addiction. In fact one might suspect that there could be a connection between all the new and different chemicals in the new or modern foods and drinks, and the modern growth in the use of cannabis, amphetamines, heroin and cocaine. In fact it is the case that diet can be very important in substance abuse, mainly through its effect on people with ADD (ADHD or ADDD).

One of our patients, who suffers from severe ADHD, was very distressed by a meal cooked with MSG, and needed extra Dexamphetamine to control his distress on the day he had the meal. One ADD patient, who had had both speed and heroin habits in the past and was currently on dexamphetamine and methadone, was quite distressed the day after eating 2 litres of ice cream as an evening meal. Another loved brightly colored, sugar coated, chocolate sweets and bought them by the kilo at a supermarket. This confectionary may have contributed to his multi-substance abuse by aggravating his ADHD, which was the main factor underlying his speed and heroin addictions. Another patient would wake up hyper-alert and unable to go back to sleep, 4 hours after drinking wine which contained preservative number 223 and would be quite distressed and aggressive the following day. He had no problems after drinking wine containing preservative number 220. It was the additive, not the alcohol, that was the problem in this case.

Most people appear to tolerate the things they fancy in the way of food and drink. However people who are substance abuse or addiction prone, or who have other signs of unusual chemistry, such as ADD or allergies, need to learn to observe any adverse feelings or functioning that they experience, in the period after consuming particular items. Even the things they crave and love may have a sting in the tail for them, causing them distress and disturbed function, and leading them to seek relief and better function, through drugs. This is a particular problem if the drugs they take to relieve their distress and dysfunction, are what caused the distress and dysfunction in the first place, as may be the case in some people taking too much caffeine, alcohol or benzodiazepines. The search for things that disturb your chemistry may be aided by observing and asking members of your family what disturbs them, as it is probably a genetic problem that runs in some families. Your partner or other family members or flatmates may help, by observing when you are disturbed, and helping you to go back over the foods and drinks you had in the previous 24 hours, that may have caused the disturbance, and need to be deleted from your diet and your shopping list or social habits.

Every substance abuse prone or addicted person should, by noticing how they feel and perform and what cravings they have, after different foods and drinks, build up:

1. A **No No** Drink List – a list of drinks that make them hyperactive, sleepless, aggressive or thick in the head and may cause them to crave drugs.

2. A **No No** Snack List – snacks that result in them feeling uncomfortable, performing poorly and being more likely to crave addictive substances.

3. A **No No** Shopping List –what not to buy when food shopping.

4. A **No No** Restaurant List – what to avoid when at a Café or Restaurant, or what Cuisines, Cafés or Restaurants to avoid altogether.

Very worthwhile help may be obtained in managing unusual chemistry and any dietary induced problems you may have, by reading everything you can on the Feingold web site www.feingold.org (Dr Ben Feingold was a Californian Allergist), or Hertha Hafer's book, The Hidden Drug Dietary Phosphate www.phosadd.com. There is also a lot of other helpful information on the internet and in other books.

DIET IS SIGNIFICANT IN TREATING HEROIN ADDICTION, ADD/ADHD, ALLERGIES AND OTHER CHRONIC CONDITIONS

By Jane Donlin (bjdonlin@ iinet.net.au) and Neil Beck

Many people, especially those who are prone to substance abuse, those who have ADD/ADHD and those who have allergies and/or other chronic conditions, are unable to tolerate certain foods.

All foods manufactured by the food industry contain one or several food additives such as preservatives, emulsifiers, lecithin, thickeners, mineral salts, colouring agents, flavours, bleaching agents, flour aerators and so forth. Every additive that goes into our food has a specific function: it improves the flavour, texture, prolongs shelf-life and suchlike.

For example preservatives prolong the shelf-life of foods; emulsifiers enhance the texture and ensure constant consistency; flavour enhancers bring out the flavour of certain foods; bleaching agents whiten flour, pasta and rice; flour aerators improve the performance of the flour in bread making; mineral salts enhance the texture of processed meats, which otherwise lose fats and juices and so on.

Some additives occur naturally such as lecithin, vitamins, minerals, sugar and salt. Salt, vinegar and sugar are the most common food preservatives and have been used to preserve meat, vegetables and fruit for centuries. Sulphur dioxide is one of the oldest naturally occurring preservatives and was used by the Ancient Greeks, Romans and Egyptians to preserve wine thousands of years ago. It is still used today (preservative number 220) to preserve wine but has many other functions as well. However, even natural additives are not healthy when used excessively or in combination with other food chemicals.

Unhealthy foods cause sensitive people to feel uncomfortable, unhappy, irritable; they perform poorly, find it difficult to concentrate, find it hard to get motivated; some become hyperactive, nervous, aggressive; others may develop headaches, itchy skin, stomach aches, nausea or allergies or feel generally unwell.

Sensitive people need to learn what foods and drinks to avoid to prevent them from experiencing these undesirable effects.

Below are lists of foods and drinks most people can consume without any problems, but which may sometimes cause serious problems for people with unusual chemistry, e.g. people with a tendency to substance abuse, addictions, emotional and social problems, eating and weight disorders, allergies and unexplained aches and pains.

Obviously we are not able to list every undesirable item available on the supermarket shelf. We have, however, attempted to list the most readily available foods which may cause the biggest problems. Given time and with practise and commonsense, most people will be in a position to recognise which foods have major adverse effects on general well-being and health.

Drinks which can cause hyperactivity, sleeplessness, aggression, which make people 'thick in the head' and may cause them to crave drugs a few hours later, include:

Soft drinks:

Cola drinks

Soda drinks

Lemonade, orange and other fizzy drinks

Fruit juice cordial containing 25% or less fruit, especially those coloured green or red

Sport drinks

High energy fizzy drinks

Chocolate flavoured milk

Strawberry flavoured milk (instant powder)

High energy milk food drinks

Soy drinks

Soluble coffee granules

Dilute all cordials 1:5 (one part cordial, five parts water)

Alcoholic drinks:

Beer, especially in large quantities

Malt beer

Wine with preservative number 223

Spirits (eg vodka, whisky and other hard liquors)

Champagne

Snacks which may make sensitive people feel uncomfortable, perform poorly and more likely to crave addictive substances, include:

Sweet Snacks:

Chocolate bars

Sugar-coated chocolate buttons

Chocolate, any kind, even white

Chocolate coated biscuits

Chocolate chip biscuits

Cream biscuits

Oatmeal biscuits

Bran or wheatmeal biscuits

Chocolate cake

Jam sponge cake (Swiss roll)

Cake glazed with icing sugar

Cheese cake

All cakes containing preservatives

Rice pudding

Lemon meringue pie

Muffins and scones (shop bought)

Doughnuts and jam balls

Glazed fruit buns

Pikelets

Waffles

Coloured popcorn

Candy and lollies

Jelly babies, jelly beans, jelly snakes

Marshmallows

Coco pops

Fruit loops

Ice-cream, dairy (shop bought)

Sweet pastries:
eg apple, berry or apricot pies
(shop bought)

Yoghurt, all types including fruit

Muesli bars

Liquorice All Sorts

Savoury Snacks:

Processed cheese

Cheese spread

Cream cheese

Cheese on toast

Cracker biscuits

Sour cream dips

Crumpets

Pies & pastries (shop bought)

Sausage rolls

Frankfurters, especially the little red ones

Ham rolls

Processed meat (ham, beef, chicken, pork) rolls

Slice of ham/cheese/egg quiche

Beef burgers (contain preservatives)

Chicken burgers (contain preservatives)

Pizza

Mixed nuts

Peanut butter sandwiches

Salted popcorn

Corn snacks

Tortilla chips

Cheese flavoured snack food (eg. potato or corn chips)

Barbecue flavoured snack food

Pizza flavoured snack food

Chicken or Beef flavoured snack food

Burger rings & cheese twisties

Instant soup mix

Two minute noodles

Things that you should think twice about before putting them on your **Shopping List** if you have unusual chemistry, include:

Sweet foods:

Ice-cream, dairy
Ice magic
Popsicles
Frozen cakes, pies & pastries
Packaged cakes & biscuits
Chocolate biscuits, all brands
Sponge cakes, with or without jam
(eg Swiss roll)
Cake mix
Christmas pudding/cake
Chocolate nut spread
Cocoa powder, drinking chocolate
Pancake mix
Instant pudding (packet-mix)
Jellies
Skim milk powder
Custard, powder & ready to use
Chocolate & fruit mousse
Yoghurt, plain & fruit
Caramel pudding, trifle
Canned fruit in thick syrup
Sweet fruit jams

Confectionary:

Chocolate bars, candy and lollies
Sugar or chocolate coated nuts
Brightly coloured chocolate buttons
Honeycomb, Turkish delight
Jelly babies, jelly snakes, jelly beans
Marzipan

Cereals:

Fruit loops
Sugar-coated cornflakes
Coco pops
Honey covered puffed wheat

Muesli bars

Savoury foods:

Frozen instant meals, e.g. lasagne, macaroni, burgers, quiches, pizzas, etc.
Instant gravies & stock powder
Sauces (packet-mix)
Instant soups (packet-mix)
Stuffing (packet-mix, sage & onion)
Ham, bologna and other cold processed meats
Frankfurters and other sausages (preservatives)
Liver paté
Bacon
Frozen pies, pastries & sausage rolls
Tomato sauce
Barbecue sauce
Soy sauce and other soy products
Mayonnaise
Margarine
Peanut butter
Frozen fish fingers
Fish cakes
Canned tuna, anchovies & herring
Canned corn beef, ham & spam
Canned soups
Canned meals (ravioli, beans & sausages, etc)
Cheese spread
Cream cheese
Mortadella
Rice, polished & easy cook
Instant noodles (two minute)
Nuts, mixed
Evaporated milk
Sweetened condense milk
Buttermilk
Coffee Mate
Instant coffee (soluble coffee granules)
Legumes - dried beans, peas & lentils
Oat bran flakes & wheatgerm
Infant cereals

Things to think twice about before ordering when at a **Café** or **Restaurant**, if you have unusual chemistry, are:

It is best to visit a Café or Restaurant where fresh foods are prepared daily on the premises.

Avoid:

All fizzy and soda drinks, especially cola
Iced coffee or chocolate
Café au lait

Sausage rolls
Quiche
Ham or bacon sandwiches/rolls
Toasted cheese & ham sandwich
Pizza
Omelette and other egg dishes
Pancakes

Chocolate mud cake
Cheese cake
Sponge cakes with cream
Muffins & scones
Sugar-coated biscuits or cakes
Ice-cream

Cuisines to avoid altogether:

All fast food outlets.
Fast foods are almost always high in fat and salt content and the meats contain preservatives like sodium nitrate (preservative number 251) or sodium phosphate (preservative number 339) to ensure a long shelf-life. These preservatives are known to cause hyperactivity, irritability and migraine headaches.

Fast food outlets include restaurants that sell:

Beef and chicken burgers, ready in three minutes
Chicken pieces & chicken nuggets
Pizzas
Chinese take-away (is very high in fat content and often has added M.S.G.)
Asian curries or other Asian cuisines
Fish & chips (high in fat & salt)
European pork or beef & gravy meals

Thick shakes
Chocolate, strawberry or caramel sundaes
Soft serves

Jane Donlin translated Hertha Hafer's book, "The Hidden Drug, Dietary Phosphate" ISBN 0-64640644-2 from German to English in the year 2000. Copies of this book in English are available from the website www.phosadd.com, by Emailing Jane at bjdonlin@iinet.net.au, or by phoning her in Australia on (08) 9497 1226.

SHARED CONSULTATION MINI MARATHONS.

Substance Abuse and ADD patients require much more frequent, regular and extended periods of healthcarer contact time, than is required by most other types of patients. However there are usually not enough appointments, and especially not enough longer appointments, available. Also people with this type of problem often miss many of their appointments or come late. For these reasons often not much progress is made and many patients get missed or lost along the way.

The problem of the need for regular extended healthcarer contact time, as well as a number of other problems, can be very effectively overcome by the use of **Shared Consultation Mini Marathons**, in place of the usual one to one consultations.

If you have three to nine patients gathered around a table and during each person's consultation, others are allowed to ask questions and to learn what they can from several consultations, instead of from just one consultation, some very positive and beneficial things start to occur, which result in individuals making much greater progress than is usual in individual one to one consultations.

The first thing is that there is usually much more energy and much more motivation and focus. The patients seem to really come alive in a group and to focus more effectively on the problems associated with Substance Abuse and the ways in which they can be dealt with.

People who have been stuck with one particular attitude, or with one way of seeing or doing things, become aware that other people see and do things differently. You will see them arguing and debating and defending their past points of view, but will also see some considering new and different ways and sometimes embracing them. People who have been bogged down or stuck for long periods, sometimes suddenly get free of the bog or the sticking point. They suddenly go over, around or under blocks which they have previously found insurmountable.

Members of the group often express opinions on solutions, suggestions or comments made by the healthcarer. They may say that this or that won't work, but suggest something else that did work for them. Individuals with real life experiences of Substance Abuse and Multiple Major Problems, sometimes teach the healthcarers, as well as other group members, very important things.

You will often see patients being very much encouraged and empowered by finding they are not alone, by finding that there are others who have, or have got through, similar difficulties to their own. They may be strengthened by the discovery that some other people have had problems even worse than theirs, but still are making it, or have made it. Companionship, support and friendship often develop, sometimes with great benefit.

In Shared Consultations healthcarers sometimes learn things about their patients that they may not have learned in a dozen individual one to one consultations. As you work with one patient, you will see in your peripheral vision actions and reactions by other patients, which would have been suppressed in the direct eyeball to eyeball interaction of one to one consultations. **There is a very real sense in which you don't fully know someone, until you have observed them in a group interacting with other people.**

Many healthcare professionals, as well as patients, may be horrified by this concept of Shared Consultations, fearing the loss of privacy and confidentiality and the possibility of loss of control. The room and the round table with four to ten chairs around it, at which I conduct my Shared Consultations, has a smaller, more standard consulting room, immediately adjoining it. All new patients are advised that when their consultation turn comes, they only have to say the word and I will immediately take them into the smaller consulting room and see them there privately. Those who take part in the Shared Consultations also observe that I do not hesitate to take a patient into the private consulting room, if an issue comes up which they do not want, or which it would not be appropriate, to discuss in the group setting.

One of the reasons some addiction patients sometimes don't like Shared Consultations is that they feel far less able to lie and cheat and manipulate the doctor in front of a group of other people, who usually know exactly what they are up to. Group consultations seem to result in more honest communication than do one to one consultations.

I just shudder when I think about the possibility of going back to only consulting by the old one to one system with Substance Abuse/ADD patients, because of the time that gets wasted, the lack of progress, the people who need to be seen that day but who can't get an appointment and the ineffectiveness and dullness so common with that type of consultation process.

Many addicts need the continuity of support, or the power to break through, of being seen every day for a few days at critical times. Also when an addict needs help, or is ready to move, they need to be seen that day or, at the latest, by the next day. The Shared Consultation System makes this possible. Patients often go backwards or relapse if they are not seen at critical times of special need. Shared Consultation Mini Marathon sessions that people can be fitted into any day of the week, can often prevent patients losing ground or relapsing. If a lot of people come on one day I have to go faster, but at least they all get seen and they don't spend soul deadening hours in the waiting room.

Some people, with (1) too many genetic problems, (2) the unresolved effects of too many past traumas, (3) too many difficulties or traumas in their present circumstances, and (4) a lack of real pleasures and satisfactions in their life, become swamped, overwhelmed, bogged down, stuck, paralysed. All they can see/hear/feel are problems. There is nothing light or bright in their life or at the end of their tunnel. Their chemistry becomes almost completely negative. They lose their cheerfulness, confidence, strength, self-esteem, ability to communicate and to do things. It can be extremely difficult to break out of this disastrous state/position with one to one consultations, but comparatively easy to do so with Shared Consultation Mini Marathons, on several days in a row.

Overwhelmed, exhausted people may need Holiday Therapy, or to be put to bed for a few days or a week under heavy sedation and constant care - Oblivion Therapy - before they are well enough to take an active part in group therapy. However they may also benefit from sitting in on a group as an observer, not saying anything or dealing with anything, but taking in some of the ideas, energy, breakthroughs and hope that usually radiates from those taking an active part in the group.

THERAPY GROUPS IN THE
TREATMENT OF HEROIN ADDICTION

Heroin addicts, many of whom suffer from Attention Deficit Hyperactivity Disorder and other disturbing conditions, have great difficulty in getting treated adequately, because of the disturbed way their brain functions and the pressures created by heroin addiction. Their sense of the passage of time is very poor so that they have difficulty in making and keeping appointments and being on time. They have difficulty in affording prescriptions and in taking medications according to the quantities and times prescribed. They have great difficulty in transport, financial management and paying bills and sometimes can't even afford a bus or train fare.

It is very difficult for a healthcare professional to get enough regular one to one consultation time with a heroin addict to give them effective treatment. The healthcare professional doesn't usually have enough time in the first place, to deal effectively with such difficult problems and then there are too many missed appointments.

Probably 90% or more of addicts do not access enough healthcare assistance to be effectively helped, through the traditional one to one consultation system. Many addicts and their families and friends are in a negative mental focus and chemical state much of the time and the things that occur during their attempts to arrange and have consultations with healthcare professionals, may increase the negativity on both sides.

An alternative to the traditional consultation system which may sometimes be better for all concerned, is **Group Therapy** where 3 to 12 addiction patients meet in a group with their healthcarers for 1 or 2 hours. It is then not a big problem if some of them come late or don't come at all. The time will still be put to good use with those who do come. If extras need help that day they can usually be fitted into the group. It can't be an intimate group where people open up deeply, but it can be very effective. The groups patients attend initially are **Shared Consultation Mini Marathons.**

More stable, intimate, confidential **Positive Therapy Groups**, that deal with deeper, more personal, more specialized issues, are arranged for patients as they make progress, become more reliable and get to enjoy, value and respect their group sessions. Many people learn things, make changes and grow more, through watching and listening to others working in therapy groups, than they do through standard one to one counselling consultations. They see and hear things from different angles. They observe other people making mistakes which they have not previously realized, or been able to admit, they are making themselves. They observe other people discovering solutions which are also relevant to them. Much more group time than individual consultation time can be provided for each person. Healthcarers often learn many valuable things about their patients from their interactions and body language in a group, which they would not learn in a one to one consultation and can therefore help these patients more.

However one to one consultations are more helpful for some problems - we need to use both methods. For most people it is probable that approximately two group sessions for every one individual conventional consultation, is likely to give the best results.

CLOSED, POSITIVE FOCUS, POSITIVE CHEMISTRY, MULTI-STRATEGY, THERAPY GROUPS

One of the most important balances in life is the balance between Your Awareness of Your Problems and Your Awareness of the Good Things in Your Life. Many people focus only on one, or the other. This gets them into serious difficulties, whether they focus only on the problems, or only on the good things.

People who focus exclusively on the problems in their life and forget about the good and happy things may become very serious, pessimistic and unhappy, losing their sense of humour and their enjoyment and love of life. They may develop mood, eating, sleeping, relationship and drug problems. They may become weakened emotionally, intellectually and physically and lose their power to solve their problems and to stay on top of life.

People who only focus on the light and bright things in their life and try to avoid awareness of problems, build up an ever increasing baggage of neglected unresolved issues, and live in an increasingly unreal world. They become less and less responsible as other people have to cover and take responsibility for the things they have neglected. This failure to deal with problems always comes at a price, usually with the loss of capability, self determination and independence, making them increasingly vulnerable. Usually, sooner or later everything becomes very complicated and difficult and they may crash or have to run away, in one way or another, from their mounting collection of untackled issues.

Some counselling and group therapy focuses too much on problems, so we try to avoid this. In Positive Therapy Groups we focus,

(1) firstly on the good things, to get the positive chemistry and energy flowing, lift our spirits and strengthen ourselves.

(2) then we face up to, analyse and resolve one single manageable problem area,

(3) and then we refocus on the positive things and get our positive chemistry going again. We encourage the group members to try to stay in that happy positive state until it is time to deal with another problem.

A more detailed explanation of what we do is as follows.

(1) Firstly we focus people's attention on the positive things in them and around them. This in turn will activate their positive chemistry - they will feel happier, more friendly, more communicative, more confident and stronger because of the chemistry which flows in their brain and body when they focus on positive things. You can change your chemistry, or that of other people, in a few moments, by changing what you are focusing on in your mind (seeing, hearing or feeling in your mind - that is remembering, thinking and imagining), or with your senses (seeing with your eyes, hearing with your ears or feeling in your body).

Some people have the habit of mostly focusing on positive things whilst others mostly focus on negative things; the first group are usually happy and positive and the second group are often pessimistic, stressed or depressed, because of the way their chemistry is changed by what they focus on.

The main thing is that you have a better life and you are stronger if your chemistry is positive. However, with depression it is the other way around. Your low brain serotonin (a chemical deficiency) causes you to focus on negative things and this in turn depresses you further. Depressed people may find it very difficult to focus on positive things, without first taking antidepressants to boost their serotonin levels.

(2) Secondly we identify and treat a currently relevant problem area, with a full armamentarium of weapons. We use Relevant Information, Cognitive Therapy, Gestalt Therapy, Transactional Analysis, Neurolinguistic Programming, Psychodrama, Common Sense or anything else that works and which the therapists are competent in.

This will focus group members on negative things and activate their negative chemistry. They will feel uncomfortable and probably will hurt, at times quite badly. However it is essential, one manageable piece at a time, to work on all the areas that are causing problems and to correct or cure them. The initial generation of positive chemistry will give group members more strength to deal with their problem issues and a reduction in their problems will in turn reduce the amount of negative chemistry these issues generate. As the ratio between Positive Focus and Positive Chemistry on the one hand and Problems, Negative Focus and Negative Chemistry on the other hand, gets better and better, somewhere along the line they will have the strength to Beat Heroin.

Encouragement, support, optimism and humour from the therapist and the group members will help greatly. Just being part of or belonging to a group can be a very positive, empowering experience. The therapist may gain insights into the patient's nature and condition through this process, which may enable helpful changes to be made in medications and other parts of the management. Insights gained during this therapy may also reveal the need for other treatments.

A highly desirable ability to have in the end, is the ability to maintain positive chemistry, even whilst focusing on and dealing with problem areas. However to do this you have to limit your problem focusing to short sharp bursts, not exceeding half an hour at a time, so that you don't overwhelm your positive chemistry and turn it into negative chemistry.

(3) Then finally we refocus on positive things again and leave group members focused as much as possible, in their mind and with their senses, on positive things, with positive chemistry flowing again, as revealed by facial expressions, voice tones and interactions. We try to teach them to live by this rhythm of mostly focusing on the positive things in their life; then as necessary, facing and resolving their problems, one manageable bit at a time; then swinging back to focus on the positive things again.

Completing The Systematic, Comprehensive, Chemical Health Record is the most reliable way of discovering an addict's Pre-existing Underlying Problems. However if well managed, these Positive Therapy Groups will probably be the most powerful method available to both discover and correct the unresolved, hidden, Pre-existing and Underlying Problems that gave rise to the addiction and that may give rise to relapses. Groups are very important.

In many cases the job is only half done until the ex addict has had extensive group therapy. By this means the ex addict may be able to turn the whole negative nightmare experience of underlying problems and addiction into a positive, by becoming a stronger, wiser and happier person than he would ever normally have been.

However, Therapy Groups are part of a bundle of strategies and will not do the job on their own, any more than medications, information or social rehab will do the job on their own.

Pacing is very important. We try to be sensitive to whether the group is flowing too quickly or whether it is going too slowly. Are people getting left behind and confused or are they getting bored and restless?

We try to **avoid doing too much**. If too much is covered it may leave group members swamped or confused and undo the good done earlier in the session. We try to monitor facial expressions and voice tones and to see, hear and feel when each patient has got/done enough and should move on or stop. When a patient has got a point clearly, it is important not to risk them losing it again, by going over it again. You can usually tell from "Ahah" facial expressions and voice tones, when someone has got the message or the solution.

The atmosphere and culture of the group is of great importance in helping to carry participants on to success. The atmosphere and culture is developed to generate positive sensations, thoughts, chemistry and interactions and to avoid negative sensations, thoughts, chemistry and interactions in the group members. The atmosphere and culture should include such things as humour, optimism, identification and highlighting of strengths, praise, camaraderie, intimacy, openness, support, goodwill, commonsense, no nonsense information, non game playing interactions, dignity and the valuing of each individual, but not intrusiveness.

Confidentiality has to be handled very skillfully. Although group therapy is very beneficial, some issues will need to be dealt with later, privately, one to one, or if there is a group co-therapist, the co-therapist may be able to take a patient from the group, into a separate room and deal with an issue on the spot.

The number in the group is critical – 3 to 12 people. **Acoustics and the seating layout** of the room are important - not too close and not too spread out.

"Heavy" consultations or group therapy, where there is too much focusing on too many problems, very little focusing on positive things and no activation of positive chemistry, but much activation of negative chemistry, may make patients worse, rather than better.

Before joining a Therapy Group each person should have their **Comprehensive Chemical Health Record completed** so that it can be referred to and added to by the therapist during and after the group meetings. It is impossible to deal with something as complicated and difficult as narcotic addiction and its Pre-existing, Underlying Factors, without keeping a comprehensive, systematic record of the history, findings and treatments and building up a complete and clear picture of the addict, his family, background and present circumstances. Trusting to memory too many patients with many problems, disorganized medical records and too many changes of healthcarers are common causes of failure in heroin clinics.

Another way of describing Positive Focus, Positive Chemistry, Multi-Strategy, Group Therapy, is

(1) Ask several group members to remember and recount to the group,

  a) Something that **made them happy** in their past life, or that **is making them happy now,** or **which they are looking forward to in the future**.

  b) **Anything they have learned** in the last few weeks or months which has made or will make their life better and happier and more how they want it to be. Then get them to congratulate themselves for discovering this information and to be grateful for the sources of this knowledge.

  c) **Anything they have done** recently, that has or will make their life better and happier and more how they want it to be. Then to thank anyone who has helped them do this thing or these things.

(2) a) Then get group members to **describe something which is spoiling their life** at present, and which they feel it is time to deal with. Then choose one group member to work on their problem.

  b) Get them to do Gestalt Therapy 2 or 3 chair work to clarify what they **really feel, think and want,** what their goals and what their time frames are, and whether they are really ready for the work and changes involved in getting what they want.

c)   Get them to consider and decide what they need to **learn**, or need to **do** and what **help**, **support** or **therapy** they need, to deal with this **one** thing.

(3) Then do therapy with them on that **one** area of difficulty, need or desire, using any information, aids or above mentioned therapies familiar to you, which are relevant. Call for input from co-workers and other group members.

Consider and ask questions about anything you have observed about them that might lead you to suspect a chemical or brainwave dimension to their condition, e.g. excessive mood swings, excessive anxiety, euphoria, depression, manic tendencies, ADHD, an overactive or underactive thyroid gland, excessive caffeine, alcohol, nicotine, sedatives or drugs, etc.

Give referrals, appointments, homework, exercises, and prescriptions as necessary. Finish with congratulations and hugs.

(4) Then work with other group members, one at a time, on their problems.

(5) Then get group members to again think about happy things from the past, the present, or which they are looking forward to in the future. Get them to see, hear, feel, smell or taste anything they have enjoyed, do enjoy or may enjoy in the future.

Teach them to practice recalling happy things, re-experiencing them as vividly as possible, whenever they have spare time, are worried or depressed, can't sleep or are tempted to go out and score drugs. Teach them to see and smell the flowers, to see and hear the birds, to pat the dog and stroke the cat, to enjoy good food and drink and music, singing, dancing, sport, reading and T.V. Teach them to give themselves things to look forward to, without living their lives in the future.

Get them focused on positive things, till their positive chemistry is flowing well and you can see it on their faces, hear it in their voices and it is apparent in their interactions. Some, who are too depressed, sad, angry, anxious etc may need medication to enable them to get started in these mental habits, but try to teach them to function in these ways without the need for nicotine, caffeine, alcohol, cannabis or other uppers or downers.

Help them to realise that a balance of Positive Focus and Solving Problems is the best way to get and keep their positive chemistry flowing, that heroin is sugar coated hell and that social and illegal drugs and abuse of prescribed drugs are not the answer.

BUPRENORPHINE OR METHADONE MAINTENANCE AS AN ALTERNATIVE TO DETOXIFICATION

Many comparatively normal people, from comparatively normal circumstances, become addicted to narcotics through such factors as a painful injury or sickness, curiosity, carelessness, peer pressure, an addicted partner, boredom, or going to nightclubs. Once they realise their mistake, it is not too difficult, using the detoxification methods described, plus naltrexone as a maintenance agent, for them to beat heroin and become drug free again.

Other people are very different. Their inner life, their brain chemistry, their psychological functioning, their social environment or life circumstances, are so disturbed and distressing that they have desperately sought relief and escape. They may have resorted to prescribed drugs, excessive alcohol or in more severe cases, may have turned to narcotics. On narcotics their life gets even worse between hits, because of the things they have to do in order to get the drug, possibly the loss of employment, home and family, perhaps jail and because of the hanging out when they can't get their next hit. It is much more helpful to think of them and call them **People With Multiple Severe Problems** rather than "addicts". "Addiction" is a great underestimation and simplification of their real situation.

Sooner or later **People With Multiple Severe Problems** nearly always come to feel very strongly the need to beat heroin and break their addiction. Their family, friends and healthcare advisers support this idea strongly - they all think the distress is due to the addiction and focus on this. They don't realise that the original problems, the **Pre-Existing Underlying Distress**, is usually still the largest part of the problem. They see the addiction as the full picture, when it is only a part of the picture. They pressure the addict to get clean. However, the addict is usually rapid cycling between pulling in two opposite directions. He wants to escape from the agony of **The Nightmare Life Between Hits**, but he craves and lives for the **Relief And Euphoria Period** each heroin hit gives him. Each hit relieves him of both his drug craving and the underlying distress that made him an addict in the first place, and replaces them with a wonderful feeling for a few hours. As the hit wears off The Nightmare Life Between Hits strikes him again. It is easy to be ambivalent and it may not be at all clear to him which way he should go with regard to his habit. He often repeatedly goes forwards then backwards.

He may come in to be detoxed and start to take an antagonist (blocker) and many who do this go on to be successful. However he may stop his blocker, sometimes even within a day or two of being detoxed, and not carry through. The family, the doctors, the law, his financial position, or desperate unrealistic hope, may have pushed him into detoxing before he was ready; then his Pre-existing Underlying problems may have caused him to seek narcotic relief again; or the craving and the deaths may have got to him. Everyone is then disgusted with him and he is likely to be disgusted with himself, which can be very damaging. He may come back and be detoxed and go onto blockers several times, especially if he is at an unstable stage of life, or if he has still got too many undiagnosed and unresolved Preexisting Underlying problems.

If multiple relapses occur, it may be that longer term maintenance narcotic addiction, using Buprenorphine or Methadone, would be better for him, than frequent repetitions of the Heroin/Detoxification/Naltrexone/Relapse Cycle, with repeated blows to self esteem, relationships, confidence and stability and with risk of overdosing. Detox followed by Naltrexone Maintenance Therapy is probably worthwhile, even if only a 6 month heroin free period follows. However if Detoxification is needed several times in a year, ongoing maintenance addiction using Buprenorphine or Methadone, has to be considered as an alternative to detoxification from narcotics, until more Preexisting Underlying problems are sorted out and there is greater clarity, adjustments stability, support and determination.

To put a comparatively normal person with a reasonable environment and only a moderate addiction onto Methadone is a tragedy, when Buprenorphine Detox and a period of blocker maintenance would fairly easily make them drug free. However the frequently repeated detox cycle may indicate serious underlying problems that still need to be dealt with and may make Buprenorphine or Methadone Maintenance Stabilisation advisable for the time being, whilst these underlying problems are searched for and dealt with more adequately. Detoxification from all narcotics will then be successful long term.

Methadone is a powerful synthetic narcotic with a number of advantages and disadvantages.

The Advantages of Methadone Include That -

(a) It does not involve injections and therefore avoids the risks of Septicaemia, Endocarditis, Hepatitis B and C and HIV from shared or dirty needles (although the use of intravenous drugs in addition to Methadone, continues in approximately 50% of cases).

(b) The addict on Methadone usually has regular contact with healthcare professionals who are trained, experienced and resourced to help people with addiction and associated problems. They also know when to refer addicts to other appropriate consultants or agencies, which may help further. However the sort of doctors and agencies that are big on Methadone are often small on helping in other ways and may have a vested interest in the addict staying on methadone and not getting better.

(c) The addict on Methadone may develop a comparative stability to his life, unlike what it was during the roller coaster existence of chasing and using heroin. This increased stability may greatly benefit him and his position in life.

(d) The addict is more likely to be able to hold down a job on Methadone than on heroin.

(e) Accidental overdosing with Methadone alone is unlikely with the usual Methadone programme. (However, using other narcotics, benzos, alcohol etc with Methadone may result in deaths in Methadone patients.)

(f) Methadone is a very effective physical pain killer and may be better than detoxification and naltrexone for the time being, when strong physical pain genuinely exists and will take some time to be investigated and controlled by other means.

(g) Methadone is now available through many Government clinics and is usually subsidised or free. This removes the need for lying, cheating, stealing, armed robbery, drug dealing and prostitution to get heroin. It reduces damage to both the addict and the rest of the community, reduces organized crime cash flow, resources and power and takes some of the pressure off overstretched law enforcement resources.

The Disadvantages of Methadone Include That -

(a) It is a very powerful drug of addiction so that the patient is still an addict and may continue to be part of the drug scene. Many addicts really dislike or even hate Methadone for reasons they may not be able to fully explain, but at least in part because they know they are still addicts, are still chemically chained down. It will be much harder for them to get off Methadone than it is to get off heroin when the time comes, as Methadone addiction is much stronger – perhaps ten times stronger – than heroin addiction. They are often very upset by the fact that they did not fully understand this before they went onto Methadone, even though most were probably told. Nevertheless, when the time is right, Methadone addiction can be beaten with Buprenorphine detox.

(b) Whilst on Methadone the addict may still crave and can still use other narcotics, and as many as 50% do. Methadone, especially as part of polydrug abuse, is still a potentially fatal substance. Some addicts who have graduated to Buprenorphine, go back to Methadone again so that they can still use heroin when they are able to get it.

(c) Unless addicts on methadone syrup clean their teeth several times a day and chew a lot of sugar-free gum, their teeth decay rapidly. They lose teeth and may require dentures which are difficult for them to get. This can greatly injure self esteem and self confidence, aggravating the whole situation. It can be devastating for a girl to know that if she smiles, she displays decayed teeth or gaps where teeth are missing - perhaps sometimes devastating enough to put her back on heroin. People on methadone for any length of time often begin to suffer severe pain from toothache and frequent dental abscesses.

(d) Addicts on Methadone are comparatively tied down as they have to report to the same pharmacist daily to get their dose. This may interfere with their job, or job seeking, or other important matters. After a few months or years they often get to hate having to go to a pharmacy every day so much that they curse the day they went on Methadone.

(e) Patients report other important problems such as severe chronic constipation, fluid retention, weight gain, drowsiness, loss of concentration, poor memory and debilitating lack of motivation. These problems can cause them to seriously regret going on to Methadone and to resent – or hate – whoever advised them to do so.

Should a particular patient stay on heroin, change to maintenance Buprenorphine or Methadone, perhaps as an interim measure, or detox altogether off all narcotics? This decision needs to be made by the addict, with full information and expert clinical assessment and consultation and perhaps with input from his family or supporters. The detox doctor needs to be an experienced and capable practitioner in social, psychological and organic medicine. He will also sometimes need to be able to obtain input from social workers, psychologists, psychiatrists, pain specialists, orthopaedic surgeons, rheumatologists and others, which can be very difficult with addicts and waiting lists and fees. Only a big hearted consultant will set aside time from a long waiting list to see addicts, who often come late or miss their appointments, may cause problems in the waiting room, often don't carry through with the recommended treatment and often don't pay their bills, because of their sickness and financial circumstances.

There needs to be flexibility and a willingness to change direction if Plan A does not work after a reasonable period and as the patient and his circumstances change. All of this is a tall order. No wonder the detox doctor doesn't always get it right first go, especially as he is often operating on the run when dealing with addicts, who often miss their appointments, or all come at once without appointments, and often have to be treated when they are ready rather than when the healthcarers are ready and have enough time.

Buprenorphine, A "New" & Better Maintenance Option Than Methadone.

Some of the advantages of Buprenorphine over Methadone are that:

(a) It is not nearly as powerfully addictive. It is a drug of addiction but not nearly as addictive as Methadone, which is by far the most addictive substance that I have worked with. Methadone withdrawal has been used as a form of torture. I doubt that Buprenorphine could ever be effectively used for this purpose.

(b) Around 50% of people on Methadone continue to use heroin or other narcotics, intermittently or regularly. They still crave the euphoria of heroin or morphine and Methadone doesn't stop them from experiencing these cravings because it is not a "blocker". On the other hand Buprenorphine is a powerful blocker as well as having moderate narcotic effects. People on an adequate dose of Buprenorphine very seldom crave or use heroin, because it both blocks nerve receptors and is a narcotic replacement chemical.

(c) It doesn't rot your teeth and make you embarrassed or frightened to smile, or cause you the agonizing toothache, which is common with people who are on Methadone for any length of time.

(d) It is not as sedating and you are therefore more normally alert, with more normal memory and powers of concentration. You remain more normally motivated and able to do things. You are more likely to be able to hold down a job, or to care properly for a family, on Buprenorphine than on Methadone.

(e) Buprenorphine does not usually cause chronic constipation, excessive fluid retention or weight gain.

(f) A dose of Buprenorphine is effective for more than twice as long as a dose of Methadone, so that most patients are not as tied down by Buprenorphine as they are by Methadone. Most can visit their pharmacy to pick up a dose of Buprenorphine every second day, rather than every day. A few can last 3 days on one dose.

(g) Some people on Methadone really hate the institutions and doctors that put them on Methadone. Sooner or later the tide may turn sufficiently strongly against Methadone that aggrieved Methadone addicts will be able to get lawyers to spec litigation cases or class actions against the doctors or institutions, who put them on Methadone without adequately trying other alternatives. This is most unlikely to happen with Buprenorphine.

There are very few disadvantages that I have been able to discover, with Buprenorphine. It may be a little more expensive than Methadone, but is still comparatively economical and affordable. There is alleged to have been minor problems, with illicit use of Buprenorphine as an alternative to heroin, but this is a small price to pay for all its benefits and this problem can be managed. A few chemically disturbed people seem unable to live without narcotics and Buprenorphine appears to be by far the least damaging alternative for these people, their families and communities.

N.U. male, 26 years.

N.U. is one of the most disturbed non-psychotic patients that I have ever seen. He was a problem from early in life and in that regard was similar to his father, who died early and had always been a difficult and troubled man. In his teen years N.U. became a big user of and then a big dealer in speed. He was quite hyperactive and violent and one of his favourite occupations was physically taking on at least two policemen at once. Eventually his mother managed to get him to a remote semi desert mining location, where she hoped he would not be able to get supplies of his drug. Unfortunately he came across a man with a big chunk of rock heroin and became a severe heroin addict.

With the greatest of difficulty we got him to see a psychiatrist who confirmed his ADHD. He missed his appointments, came very late, or visited the psychiatrist without an appointment, but eventually made it. At first he was prescribed Ritalin, but tried to shoot it up. The psychiatrist then prescribed dexamphetamine, but he used the full month's supply in a week. When he ran out he was beside himself until his next prescription became due and I often didn't think he was going to survive. Eventually things improved, with dexamphetamine dispensed regularly in small amounts.

He then moved around from city to city and to some country areas, with various problems arising, including relapses to heroin and to speed. Then I managed to get him onto Buprenorphine. Now he takes 32mg of Buprenorphine every day, never misses and takes nothing else, legal or illegal. Although he really needs dexamphetamine as well, that is too difficult for him to manage. Although it would help him if he were able to take other additional psychotropic medications, he is now well enough to live quite a reasonable life on his four Buprenorphine tablets each day. He is the best he has ever been in his life and he, his family and we agree that he should stay on long term maintenance Buprenorphine. There is great relief all round and it is saving the taxpayer a small fortune.

SOME PRACTICAL SOCIAL, PSYCHOLOGICAL & GENERAL FACTORS

Whilst medications and doctors are important in the treatment of narcotic addictions, there are extremely important social, psychological and general factors which also need to be carefully considered. Drug addiction is a chemical, but also a social and a psychological illness. It would be much more helpful if narcotic users were thought of and called **People With Multiple Serious Problems** rather than simply "addicts". "Addict" is usually a great simplification and underestimation of the narcotic user's predicament. If addiction was their only problem, most narcotic users could be permanently cured without too much difficulty. In real life most have multiple problems, at least some of which need to be discovered and resolved so that their burden can be reduced, before medicine can rid them of their addiction on a lasting basis.

(a) **Support** Many **People With Multiple Serious Problems** are in trouble, at least in part, because they did not have adequate support in especially difficult or traumatic periods of their past life. Some of them are people who lack skills in getting the support they need, or who put supporters off.

Narcotic addiction is destructive, dangerous and very hard to beat. Therefore, getting off narcotics is a time when you need all the support you can get from family, friends and health care professionals. You may have hurt, ripped off or alienated some of these people. You need, if possible, to get them back on your side. Go back to them and if appropriate, make amends for past mistakes and ask for their renewed love and support. Tell them you are going to give detox your best shot and that you need their help. Addicts who have good supporters and a strong support system have a better chance of beating heroin than those who don't.

(b) **General Health** You need to have treatment for any general health problems that have helped to drag you down into addiction.

If you got onto heroin to try to escape from the suffering of depression, then you must get the depression (or bipolar) problem treated. Otherwise there will be a strong pressure for you to go back onto heroin, if you get depressed again.

If you got onto heroin because of pain in your back, neck, head or anywhere else, from an industrial or a motor vehicle accident, or a painful physical illness, you must have this problem assessed and treated, or you will be at risk of going back onto heroin. The pain will come back when you stop the heroin, unless you clear up the cause. This will make it difficult for you to stay clean.

If you got onto heroin because of personal distress resulting from a family breakup, a death or other tragedy in the family, rape, sexual or physical abuse, loneliness, jail, immigration, war experiences or some other traumatic experience or situation and you have never talked about this problem with anyone, or not had proper counseling about it, you must first share this problem with someone. After sharing it you must then get counselling to help you overcome the disturbance it has caused in you.

You need to confront your problems with some suitable counsellor, for at least one session each week, until those problems no longer trouble you. Over time and with effective counselling, there is nothing you can't recover from, or come to terms with. Unresolved problems tend to weaken you and allow you to be pushed back to using heroin if new problems, crises or bad situations develop. You need to face, deal with and get rid of all your old problems so that you can devote all your strength to beating any new problems that might arise.

ADD, anxiety, panic attacks, sexual identity conflict, violent destructive outbursts, epilepsy and psychosis are some of the other health problems that need to be looked for and dealt with, if found.

Try to work out where, how and why your general health problems helped to get you onto heroin. Then resolve the causes of these general health problems, so that those problems won't be there to push you back to using again, once you are clean.

Try to build up your general fitness also. This will boost your physical and mental strength, self-esteem and confidence and help you to beat heroin. Exercise and sunlight can be of great value in beating heroin just walking for half an hour each day can be enough to work wonders.   Paying attention to diet and sleep is very important.

Addiction nearly always occurs as the result of multiple factors or causes. You won't get rid of all of these in one quick, grand effort, but you will win if you keep on finding and fixing the factors, one small manageable bit at a time.

(c) **General Life Needs** We all need regular exercise, good food, adequate sleep, a reasonable home, good friends or family, non-damaging fun or pleasure, some degree of structure and probably some work or duties, in our life. If you are an addict, with multiple problems, you need these things even more than other people need them, but are more likely to be lacking in some of them.

Addicts are often very focused on sleep (although often at odd times), but not on exercise or diet. It is essential to get regular exercise even if it is only to walk for half an hour a day in the fresh air and the sunlight. This will, in particular, help with sleeping and general strength, a sense of well-being, confidence, self-esteem and appetite. It is essential to have good food even if it is only fresh fruit and vegies, milk and wholemeal bread. Don't just live on fatty, salty take-away foods, cigarettes, coffee, cola drinks and TV. You can't fight anything if you are unfit, malnourished and inadequately rested – especially something tough like heroin.

There is a strong association between drug addiction, mental health problems and sleep disturbance, in particular, sleeping in the day and staying up at night. It is essential to try to get back to a pattern of sleeping at night and staying awake and up and about during the day, with minimal sedatives taken during the day. Sedatives such as Valium and Serepax taken during the day make it harder for you to sleep at night.

Do you have a reasonable place to live in and family or clean friends to be with? Do you have satisfying and rewarding work? Do you have fun and non-damaging pleasure in your life? Do you have at least some structure or routine to your life, or is it all over the place, total chaos?

(d) <u>**Varying Social Attitudes   to Brain Affecting Chemicals**</u>   There is a great variation in attitudes toward brain affecting drugs and medications amongst different nationalities, communities, families and individuals. Some readily accept the social drugs caffeine, nicotine, alcohol and perhaps marijuana, whilst others don't. Some readily accept prescribed tranquillisers and sleeping medications whilst others don't. Some happily accept both groups of chemicals and some are very negative about both groups of chemicals.

It is valuable for a person troubled by drug addiction to review the attitude towards drugs and medications within his family and social groups, amongst his friends and work mates and in his community and his country. The attitude of those around him was probably one of the factors which influenced him towards drugs. It may help him to beat drugs if he withdraws from some of these influences, once he has worked out which, if any, are leading him astray. New friends, groups, workplace or a new community with different attitudes to drugs, may make a great difference.

There is a common cultural attitude, especially amongst drug/medication pro people, and including some medical, nursing and other healthcare workers, that if someone is unhappy or suffering, you must give them something to put in their mouth - a drink, some food, some medicine or a drug. Although you have to take responsibility for your own drug consumption, your supporters or helpers may be making your condition worse, whilst everybody thinks they are really assisting you, through what they give you to put in your mouth. Often, but not always, doing nothing, or sharing your thoughts and feelings, exercise, sunlight and fresh air may be more helpful than a "do something" or a "do something quick" compulsion, which results in something going into your mouth. Often the "do something quick" attitude of a helper or supporter is a sign of anxiety on their part. They may be upset and destabilised by the suffering and tragedy of a situation. Past experience may mean they know how difficult the problem is, have an excessive sense of responsibility for fixing it and feel very pressured to do something.

Addicts often apply great pressure in these situations, shifting responsibility and making demands. Everyone needs to take a few deep, steady breaths, remain calm and look carefully for causes and solutions, rather than stampeding. It takes great wisdom, strength and some relaxation skills, (e.g. steady breathing) to know when to do nothing and to then do nothing, until it is clear which actions will really help and which actions may be harmful and that the timing is right. Especially when you are dealing with strong chemicals. It is doubly difficult to hold back if the patient can just go somewhere else and readily get the chemicals they want.

Sometimes addicts have very conflicting, irrational and unhelpful attitudes to chemicals. They may shoot up narcotics or speed, but absolutely refuse to take antidepressant medication or dexamphetamine, which are essential in treating the underlying problems, in some cases. Addicts tend to make snap decisions about things. Their snap decisions about what medicines they will or will not take can cause them additional months or years of suffering and delay their recovering from an addiction.

(e) **The Almost Universal Assumption That Everyone Responds To Brain Affecting Chemicals In The Same Way, Is Wrong** There is great individual variation in responses to any brain affecting chemicals we may take or use. It depends on your individual chemistry - your chemical production and your chemical break down/excretion systems, as to what effect a particular chemical may have on you.

People are chemically different - sometimes very different. Some take sleeping capsules at breakfast time each day because they help wake them up! Others take amphetamines to get calm and sleep better. (If that happens to you, get checked out for ADHD.) One small 42kg girl took 4 Mogadons and 4 to 10 Rohypnols (not supplied by me) at bedtime and still couldn't sleep.

One person may be able to drink alcohol or take tranquillisers and sleeping tablets freely and have very few problems. Another person may suffer from troublesome anxiety, sleeplessness, phobias or other unpleasant and unhelpful after effects, following consumption of moderate or even small amounts of alcohol and Benzodiazepines. This difficulty may occur in individuals or may run in families. Several members or generations of one family may have chemical problems, which may be the same or may vary from person to person. It can be of great value for addicts to carefully observe their own individual responses to the various drugs they take. Don't only take notice of how you feel at the time of consumption, but also of how you feel and perform a few hours later, or in the early hours of the morning or on the day following consumption. Don't think only of the immediate pleasure or satisfaction a drink or a pill or a shot may give you, but think of any unpleasant and unhelpful reactions you may have three hours later, or during the night, or next day. Don't be put off because most other people seem to get a different reaction to the reaction you get – sense and trust what you really feel yourself. Also observe any unusual reactions other members of your family may have to various chemicals in case this has relevance for you.

Some people's chemical system produces a **chemical rebound** after drug consumption. The pleasurable, calming or stimulating feelings which people may experience during and shortly after taking alcohol or "benzos", may be followed some time later by a **rebound** period of being excessively alert, hypersensitive, irritable, aggro and feeling sorry for themselves. (This may sometimes be a reaction to the preservatives or other chemicals in the drink rather than a reaction to the alcohol). There are happy drunks but there are also sad drunks and there are aggro, mean and nasty drunks and the differences are probably more chemical than psychological. There are calm "benzo" users, but some "benzo" users are still not calm, even when they are taking doses high enough to make them drugged and drowsy. A vicious cycle and a chronic state may develop if you take increasing amounts of alcohol or "benzos" to dampen down the nasty **rebound** stage. You need to avoid the trap of trying to treat the **rebound** with the chemical that caused it. Especially avoid taking increasing amounts and increasing the **rebound**, when trying to fix it. You may then get desperate and reach for the big H (heroin) or the big R (rohypnol) to settle it all down or blot it all out with disastrous consequences. Less drugs or no drugs at all - not more drugs – is sometimes the way to go if you want to stop feeling so bad and want to feel good again.

The almost universal assumption that everyone responds in the same way to drugs and medications, can be serious. Individuals need to take drugs and medications differently and they need to be treated differently by the doctors who prescribe for them. Again and again small teenage females, weighing less than 45 kilos, run into side effects from their medications, because they have been given the same dose as is given to an 90 kilo older male, when half the dose would have been much more appropriate.

Unusual or abnormal chemistry and reactions to chemicals are much more common among drug addicts than in the general community. Addicts need to observe themselves and their responses to chemicals very carefully. One of the causes of difficulty in beating drugs is unrecognized, unusual or abnormal chemistry.

"Unusual Chemistry" appears to be a problem for 10 to 20% of the total population, but amongst Addicts it is probably nearer 90%.

(f) **Misguided, Desperate and Poison People**   You not only need to gather your supporters around you, but you also need to avoid, escape from or throw out the people and the groups which helped to drag you down and who will drag you down again if you are not on guard against them.

In particular, you have to get away from all users and dealers. It is a great mistake to live in the same home or building as a user or a dealer. Even living in the same street as a dealer may be a problem. Never allow users or dealers to come into your home. If they ring you, hang up and don't even start to speak to them. They can tell from your voice tones and what you say whether you are starting to weaken. They will push you over the line if they can. Try changing your phone number. If they come to your door, don't even open it. However nice or "friendly" they seem to be, they ring or come for only one reason - to get you back onto drugs in order to make money out of you. They want you as another chook in their battery to lay another golden egg for them every day. They are usually very cunning and know exactly how to get to you even with brief contact.

You must avoid going to places where there will be users or dealers. If you have a family with users or dealers in it, then you must find ways to avoid them until they are clean. They will certainly make it easier for you to slip back if you manage to get off the narcotics. Many people who get off heroin, go back to it because of contact with users and dealers. Above all, avoid "friendly", "kind", "understanding" dealers - they are the most dangerous of all - even if they are old friends of many years' standing. Their "friendliness" is utterly hypocritical and cynical. They are wolves in sheep's clothing. They pretend to be **friendly** in order to help get you back onto **deadly** drugs!!

Most dealers are, underneath, desperate people, subject to many pressures and in great need of your money and support or agreement or acquiescence. They are in deep trouble themselves and they want you to be in deep trouble with them. They will do almost anything to make a sale or recruit a new customer so you must avoid them like the plague.

Never deal in drugs, however desperately you need the money. People who deal almost always become serious users sooner or later, often developing extreme habits, probably because of the company they keep and the pressures they experience, as well as the ready access to, and affordability of, bulk drugs.

You must also try to minimise contact with people who criticise you or run you down. They weaken your self esteem and sap your confidence and strength. Try to stay close to people who are positive and warm towards you and who build up your self esteem, confidence and strength; but not warm people who are also weak or unwise, who go along with everything you want or demand or do, including things which are damaging to you. A kind but weak and indulgent friend, partner, parent or doctor may be your downfall. The people who will help you most are likely to be warm and positive towards you, but also wise, firm, strong and disciplined.

(g) <u>**When You Leave An Institution**</u>   Because of their activities in getting sufficient money to support their drug habit, many addicts end up in jail or other institutions. It is of great value to start taking Naltrexone a few days before you leave an institution where you have detoxed the hard way, because drugs and medications were not available.   If you don't do this, it is possible that you will be back on heroin on the same day that you leave the institution. All your withdrawal suffering will then be wasted.   Speak to any doctor or authority at the institution that you can, about getting onto naltrexone.   If they are not able to help you, get family or friends to beg, borrow or buy naltrexone tablets through Next Step, a heroin clinic, or from a pharmacy with a script from a G.P.   Start with a quarter of a tablet each morning, at least 3 or 4 days before leaving the institution, then increase to half or a whole tablet each morning before you get out. If you can't start the naltrexone before you leave the institution, start it on the day that you leave. Go straight to a clinic or a doctor on your way home from the institution. Keep taking the naltrexone daily for preferably one to two years, whilst you consult with doctors, counselors, clinics etc to find out why you became an addict in the first place, and resolve those preexisting underlying causes that led to your addiction in the first place.

Ten or fifteen percent of people can't tolerate a whole naltrexone tablet every day. They may get nausea or diarrhea, or be over stimulated. If this happens to you try half a tablet daily.

(h) <u>**Other Social & Psychological Consultants**</u>   It is often beneficial to have assessments, treatment and counselling from a psychologist, a psychiatrist, a social worker, a counsellor etc and this should be discussed with the doctor doing the detoxification as he/she may not be qualified to deal with some of your issues and may   need to give you referrals.   If possible, you need to develop a long term, happy relationship with at least (1) one mental health professional, (2) one G.P. and (3) one or two lay counsellors or groups. This enables you to get advice as necessary and to have someone to be able to turn to quickly for support in a crisis. It is tempting for a detox doctor to try to handle all the psychosocial issues themselves, (most of us have God Complexes!) but few are qualified or have sufficient time to do this part of the work as well as is required, for someone as complex as most drug troubled people are.

Some addicts are good at gathering helpful supporters and a strong support system around them.   Others just alienate supporters and drive them away, or attract the wrong sort of supporters – people who are useless or worse than useless and do harm.   Gathering good support around you is something you can learn to do if you realise its importance and put your mind to it. Observe how people you know who have good support, manage it. You will have a much better chance of beating heroin if you do learn to find and keep good (not bad) supporters.

A SUMMARY OF THE MEDICATIONS WHICH ARE SOMETIMES USED TO HELP BEAT HEROIN

While it would be great for addicts to get off and keep off heroin, without the use of other chemicals, this is rarely possible and people who talk about achieving it, put addicts at risk. The aim in the short term must be to make addicts less tortured, volatile and unstable and more able to function adequately and safely; in part by moving them from chemicals which give relief from their underlying problems, but which are damaging and dangerous, to chemicals which give relief but cause less danger and damage. Over time, as an addict moves from a sick and distressed, stormy and chaotic existence to a more stable and healthy state and lifestyle, and as new and better methods of diagnosis and treatment of the underlying problems are developed, less and less chemicals should be needed. In the meantime, the more an addict and his family and friends know about and understand the medications that can help in beating heroin, the sooner and surer he will beat heroin, the less medications he will need to take, the less side effects he will get from the medications and the less likely he will be, to relapse to heroin.

There are 6 main ways in which medications can help in beating heroin. They are **(1)** by giving immediate relief, **(2)** by helping stabilise the patients' mood and activity levels, **(3)** in preparing for detoxification, **(4)** in detoxification, **(5)** in withdrawal distress management and **(6)** by helping to prevent short or long term relapse. I am providing a long list rather than a short list of medications so that readers will know where everything fits in - not because these medications are always needed. Many of them will usually **not** be needed, but there will be less suffering and failure if full knowledge about all the possibilities, allows the treatment to be tailored more exactly to suit each person and situation.

1. IMMEDIATE RELIEF MEDICATIONS.

It is very strategic for a heroin clinic to give people who come to that clinic an immediate substantial reduction in their various forms of suffering – preferably on the first day that they present. Heroin addicts suffer greatly and the word out around the traps should be that those who are suffering can expect immediate help and early relief, if they go to the heroin clinic. Heroin addicts should feel that going to the clinic will provide them with quicker, cheaper and better relief than contacting their dealer. The heroin clinic should not be their last port of call, which they only go to in desperation, when they have already done great damage, have totally drained all their resources and can't even afford a bus fare or a prescription.

The clinic should provide **IMMEDIATE RELIEF:-**

(a) FROM HANGING OUT, by giving as necessary -

(i) Buprenorphine – half to 1mgms, hourly for 3 hours to start with, to help reduce the hot and cold sweats, arm, leg and back aches, gut cramps, vomiting and diarrhoea and craving. Buprenorphine is the best immediate relief medication. However if introduced in larger doses, too rapidly, a **small** proportion of patients will vomit badly, suffer Precipitated Withdrawal, severe headaches or occasionally asthma. In 95% of addicts there will have been no adverse reaction within 2 hours of their first 2 mg of buprenorphine. They can then suck 4 mg every 2 hours until their symptoms have subsided satisfactorily. They should probably not suck more than 16 mg in the first 24 hours.

(ii) Panadeine Forte, Doloxene, or Digesic, plus Vioxx, Celebrex or Surgam, when Buprenorphine is not available, relieve the aches, pains and some of the hanging out. If early detoxification and administration of naltrexone is anticipated, then the Panadeine, Doloxene and Digesic should be avoided – they are only recommended if Buprenorphine can't be obtained, as they are narcotics and not compatible with naltrexone.

(iii) Clonidine in correct amounts helps reduce the hanging out. However too much lowers the blood pressure and causes drowsiness or fainting. Usually half a tablet should be taken every four to six hours and a whole tablet at bedtime. Once the effects and side effects on this dosage have been determined, the dose can be adjusted.

(b) FROM ANXIETY, which can be relieved with Oxazepam, Diazepam, Epilim, Serotonin Boosters (SSRI's), Doxepin, Amitriptyline or Pericyazine. Benzo Tranquillisers should be used as **little** as possible, but are of value in some cases. They should only be given where really necessary and should be weaned off as soon as possible because of easy development of dependence on them.

(c) FROM INSOMNIA, which is often the worst form of suffering that heroin addicts experience during withdrawal. I prefer to give 2 or 3 x 25mgm Doxepin, (which are long lasting) early in the evening, e.g. 7.00p.m. followed by 10-50mg of Temazepam (fast acting) at bedtime. The Temazepam may be repeated during the night but the Doxepin should not be. Neither of these types of sleepers are likely to give a satisfactory result without the other, Doxepin being good at keeping people asleep but not so good at putting them to sleep and Temazepam being good at putting people to sleep, but not so good at keeping them asleep. The combination often does an excellent job, putting people to sleep and then keeping them asleep. Patient resistance to accepting these medications instead of Flunitrazepam, (which they are often desperate for) is often due to poor results in the past. This is often due to either long acting or short acting sleepers being given on their own, without the other, smaller doses being given, or slow acting sleepers being given too late in the evening.

The doses usually given to non-addicts are unlikely to be of much value with heroin addicts during the withdrawal phase. However it should always be remembered that as long as a person is taking these sleeping medications they are not getting natural, normal, fully beneficial sleep. They need to be weaned off sleepers as soon as possible, the Benzos going first. The use of the Immediate Relief Medications, especially Buprenorphine, will greatly reduce the need for sleepers.

Flunitrazepam very seldom if ever does more good than harm. It should never be given without first determining whether the patient has had it before and, if so, whether they had adverse reactions such as aggressiveness, violence and destructiveness, amnesia, going out and scoring heroin or committing armed robbery. Flunitrazepam should never be given unless there will be very strict and strong supervision of the number of tablets taken, when they are taken and of the safety of the patient and others around them, for 8 or 9 hours after they are taken.

(d) **FROM THE WITHDRAWAL SYMPTOMS** of gut cramps, vomiting and diarrhoea, if this is not controlled by the medications already mentioned. Buscopan, Maxalon, Ondansetron, Imodium or Octreotide may be used according to the symptoms and the circumstances.

2. STABILISATION MEDICATIONS.

Heroin addicts are often very unstable and suffer distressing swings in mood, activity, motivation and behaviour. The anxiety and insomnia medications mentioned above will help in the stabilisation process. However there are some medications which are particularly valuable in stabilising distressed and distressing addicts.

(a) The **MOOD STABILISERS** Epilim (valproate), Tegretol (carbamazepine), Clonazepam and Lithium will level out significant swings and have a very beneficial effect in improving sleep patterns - they are often much more useful than the usual Benzos, or may be very good in combination with reduced Benzo dosages. They seem to have particular value in hyperactive patients who have features of ADHD, manic-depressive tendencies, violent outbursts or rage and in those who can't sleep, even with a bucketful of Benzos. Usually approximately 500 mgs of Epilim morning and 1000 mgm in the evening, Tegretol CR 400mg, 1 tablet morning and evening or Lithium 450 to 500mgms morning and evening, will be satisfactory dosages to start with, but adjustments will then be needed according to patient weight, responses and blood levels. The blood should be checked regularly, to maintain correct levels. Clonazepam is a Benzo and more likely to be abused but is good for getting situations under control quickly in the early stages. Epilim has the least side effects (but it can cause weight gain) and Lithium is usually the most powerful. Blood tests for liver, thyroid and kidney function should be done and followed up carefully if abnormal.

(b) **SEROTONIN BOOSTERS (SSRI ANTIDEPRESSANTS)** such as Efexor XR, Avanza and Cipramil are very useful in stabilising people who have anxiety, panic disorder, or a depressive tendency, or who deny they have a depressive tendency but who have depressed facial appearances, voice tones and behaviour. Depending on body weight, they should start with half or one tablet each morning, increasing to one or two tablets after 2 weeks, if the result has not been satisfactory and there have been no side effects. They should continue on that dose until they have been on the medication for 4 to 6 weeks in total. If the result is not satisfactory by that time, then they should be switched to a different Serotonin Booster, after a brief wash out period. A few people have to try up to half a dozen different antidepressants before they find one which is effective for them. They need to stay on the antidepressant which is most effective for them for a minimum of 6 to 12 months, until they have been mentally strong and their heroin problem has been stable for at least 6 or 8 months.

Although these medications are usually called antidepressants, it would be better if they were called Serotonin Boosters as by boosting serotonin levels, they also help greatly with anxiety, panic attacks and brain function generally. Antidepressant is too narrow a term to describe them accurately.

(c) **STIMULANT THERAPY** It is very important to determine whether an addict suffers from ADD (ADHD or ADDD). If they do, their stabilisation will be greatly assisted by Methylphenidate (Ritalin) or Dexamphetamine. Without these medications, ADD sufferers will continue to be unstable and will probably relapse to street amphetamines and then to heroin fairly quickly. About 50% of heroin addicts are ADD sufferers. Heroin addiction and ADD may be comorbid conditions but usually it is the ADD that leads to the substance abuse. The diagnosis and then treatment of ADD with stimulant therapy in childhood reduces the risk of substance abuse in adolescence by 85%. If the diagnosis of ADD in a heroin addict is missed and stabilisation with stimulant therapy is not achieved, permanent escape from heroin will be very difficult. If stimulant therapy is hard to get, as it often is, Epilim as described above, can be a very helpful interim measure for ADHD. It is usually about 30% as effective as dexamphetamine or Ritalin.

If the addict is self medicating with large irregular intravenous doses of street speed and legal Dexamphetamine cannot be obtained, he could obtain black market Dexamphetamine instead of speed and take it orally, regularly, every morning and lunchtime, at whatever regular dose stabilises him best. Of course it is much better to do things legally but this is very slow and sometimes nearly impossible for addicts and black market Dexamphetamine is far safer and cheaper than black market speed or heroin.

Addictions may mask ADD but it is usually possible to tell from the early childhood and school history, when to suspect this condition. Dexamphetamine is so effective and essential in the stabilization of ADD/Addiction patients that, with due caution in possible manic or non drug psychosis cases, a small trial of Dexamphetamine should be given sooner rather than later when ADD is a possibility.

3.   **PREDETOX MEDICATIONS**.

Prior to Rapid Detox or Incremental (Stepped) Rapid Detox (which treatments I now never use), the **IMMEDIATE RELIEF** and **STABILISATION MEDICATIONS** should be given as indicated above. The **IMMEDIATE RELIEF** and the **STABILISATION** provided should allow the patient to become calmer and clear enough to be sure which they really want; to be detoxed from heroin, to go onto methadone or buprenorphine maintenance, or to stay on heroin for the time being. This decision should not be rushed or pressured, or made whilst they are in a desperate state and position. This preparation period is of great importance and should occur even if considerable amounts of Buprenorphine, Codeine or Doloxene and sleepers are needed to give a breathing space for decision making.

If the desire to detox is clear and definite, SPEEQE Detox, Home Detox, Incremental (Stepped) Rapid Detox or Rapid Detox can be chosen, according to the circumstances. (These days I always use SPEEQE Detox as it is so Safe, Painless, Effective, Easy, Quick and Economical and provides such immediate results and relief). Predetox Medications, which will reduce suffering and complications, and increase the chances of success, should then be given before, during and after withdrawal of the drug of addiction, according to the treatment plan. They include:

(a) CLONIDINE (CATAPRES) to reduce withdrawal symptoms.

(b) BUPRENORPHINE
Buprenorphine is a synthetic narcotic, which can be used as a stepping stone from heroin or from methadone, to a narcotic free state. It can also be used as a maintenance medication replacement for methadone, over which it has many

advantages. The Buprenorphine is given to enable other narcotics to be stopped and then, because Buprenorphine is much less addictive than other narcotics and has a narcotic blocking effect, detoxification can follow with much less difficulty. Its use during the stormy periods of change greatly facilities detox.

(c) GUT MEDICATIONS
Maxalon, Imodium and Buscopan help with withdrawal vomiting, diarrhoea and gut pains.

(d) MUSCULO – SKELETAL ACHE & CRAMP MEDICATIONS
Can give great relief e.g. Surgam or Vioxx for aches and Quinine Bisulphate for arm and leg cramps.

(e) TRANQUILLISERS & SEROTONIN BOOSTERS
To calm anxiety and agitation e.g. Serotonin Boosters, Benzos, Pericyazine.

4. DETOXIFICATION MEDICATIONS.

(a) NALOXONE (NARCAN) and

(b) NALTREXONE (REVIA)
displace narcotics from the receptors in the central nervous system. Narcan has the advantage that the withdrawal effects it produces are very much less uncomfortable than the withdrawal effects produced by naltrexone and only last a much shorter time. It is therefore usual to give narcan IVI, IMI or S/C, before the oral naltrexone. However Narcan only lasts for half an hour. Naltrexone has the advantage that it gives a much longer receptor blockage effect. Once a patient has been detoxed with narcan, naltrexone is much more suitable as a maintenance medication, as its effects last at least 24 hours.

5. WITHDRAWAL MANAGEMENT MEDICATIONS.
These medications are given as necessary to reduce the suffering and side effects of narcotic withdrawal, which occur with assisted detoxification, but usually not with Buprenorphine detoxification. They include:

(a) CLONIDINE to reduce withdrawal symptoms generally.

(b) BUPRENORPHINE to reduce withdrawal symptoms generally.

(c) MAXALON to reduce nausea and vomiting.

(d) ONDANSETRON to reduce nausea and vomiting.

(e) **OCTREOTIDE** to reduce diarrhoea.

(f) **IMODIUM** to reduce diarrhoea.

(g) **BUSCOPAN** to reduce gut cramps.

(h) **QUININE BISULPHATE** to reduce cramps in the muscles of the limbs and trunk.

(i) **VIOXX, CELEBREX OR SURGAM** to reduce general musculo-skeletal aches & pains.

6. **MAINTENANCE MEDICATIONS.**

(a) **NALTREXONE**
  (i) As long as an ex addict takes his naltrexone every day, he will not have a heroin problem again.

  (ii) Naltrexone stops craving for narcotics and it stops narcotics from having any effect if they are used, once the right dose of naltrexone is found. The correct dose is usually 1 tablet each morning, but it may be a half or a quarter of a tablet or one and a half or two tablets. The correct dose is a dose that is large enough to stop craving but small enough to minimize side effects to the point where they are not likely to cause the patient to stop his naltrexone altogether.

  (iii) If an ex addict's Pre-existing Underlying Problems that caused him to use heroin in the first place, are not discovered and dealt with, he will be in great danger of stopping his naltrexone and going back to heroin quite quickly. The sooner his Pre-existing Underlying Problems are discovered and the more effectively they are dealt with, the more likely the ex-addict is to take his naltrexone and the sooner the naltrexone can be safely weaned off.

  (iv) If he stops his naltrexone in the first year and his Pre-existing Underlying Problems have not been resolved, there is a 90-95% chance of relapse to heroin.

  (v) If he relapses to heroin for 3 days or less, then the naltrexone can usually be quickly reintroduced. Buprenorphine should be taken for 2 or 3 days. 1.x 50mgm tablet of naltrexone should be crushed in 2 litres of water or cordial and shaken well. 24 to 48 hours after the last heroin use, 40mls (half a small glass), of this mixture should be drunk and this should be repeated in two hours. If no withdrawal reaction occurs, then 40mls at a time can be drunk regularly until the whole 2 litres is finished or there is a withdrawal reaction.

If even a mild withdrawal reaction occurs, more Buprenorphine should be given and the naltrexone should be stopped for 12 hours then recommenced. This process can be repeated until the whole 2 litres has been drunk. Then half, one or one and a half tablets per day can be commenced.

(vi) An important cause of stopping naltrexone is that at least 10 - 20% of people who take it get gut or nervous side effects and at least 1% cannot tolerate it at all. They may get loss of appetite, nausea or diarrhea or they may become anxious, shaky and have difficulty sleeping. These problems can usually be overcome by crushing a naltrexone tablet and putting it in 2 litres of water, cordial or juice, shaking it well then drinking a glass full twice a day, increasing gradually until a dosage is reached where narcotic craving is substantially reduced and side effects are not sufficient to cause the patient to stop his naltrexone altogether. People who don't want to take any naltrexone at all, regardless of the reason they give, may still be wanting to keep open the option of occasional heroin shots and may need more work done on their Pre-existing, Underlying Problems.

(b) SSRI'S (SEROTONIN BOOSTERS)
Should be continued as stabilisers for at least six to twelve months after detoxification, and sometimes for years.

(c) MOOD STABILISERS (EPILIM, TEGRETOL, CLONAZEPAM & LITHIUM
Should be continued as long as is necessary and then very slowly weaned off, but   increased again if instability starts to re-emerge.

(d) STIMULANT THERAPY (RITALIN, DEXAMPHETAMINE)
Should be given for ADD if ADD is a part of the addict's Pre-existing, Underlying Causes. It should be continued as long as is necessary, in conjunction with other treatments such as Individual, Group and Family Therapy, Educational Assessment and Development, Diet, EEG Biofeedback and other developing treatments.

None of the maintenance medications should be stopped abruptly. All should be weaned off gradually at the appropriate time. If during the weaning process problems start to become apparent again, go back to the last dose that seemed to control the situation.

IN MY EXPERIENCE THE MOST VALUABLE MEDICATIONS IN BEATING HEROIN ARE VARIOUS COMBINATIONS OF BUPRENORPHINE, EPILIM (VALPROATE), SEROTONIN BOOSTERS, DEXAMPHETAMINE/RITALIN AND DOXEPIN. UNFORTUNATELY WE ARE HAMPERED IN OUR EFFORTS TO HELP ADDICTS BEAT HEROIN, BY THE REGULATIONS APPLYING TO BUPRENORPHINE, DEXAMPHETAMINE AND RITALIN. THESE REGULATIONS PROBABLY REFLECT THE FACT THAT THE PEOPLE RESPONSIBLE FOR THEM, MOSTLY DO NOT CURRENTLY WORK WITH ADDICTS ON A DAILY BASIS, IN TODAY'S REAL LIFE SITUATIONS.

A COMPREHENSIVE BUNDLE OF STRATEGIES FOR BEATING HEROIN ADDICTION

Beating Heroin is a very difficult task. Whenever you have a very difficult task you are most likely to succeed if you break it down into manageable parts; attack it in many different ways; and are persistent and keep coming back for another try; even when you have setbacks. The strategies listed are for individuals, communities and States who are endeavouring to beat heroin.

1. An Adequate Anti-drugs Media Campaign & Treatment Promotion Campaign, With Phone Numbers To Ring.

2. Easy Access To Immediate Treatment & Immediate Relief, With Minimal Delays & Obstacles.

3. Groups & One To One Consultations Of A User Friendly Nature, Seven Days A Week And Evenings.

4. An Emphasis On Continuity Of Care, Communication Skills, Rapport, Respect And No Game Playing, Between Health Care Workers & Addicts.

5. Clarification Of The Patient's Thoughts & Feelings & Confirmation & Reinforcement That He/She Definitely Wants To Leave The Drug Scene And Be Drug Free.

6. The Development Of Addict Confidence In The Knowledge, Systems, Skills, & Genuine Interest Of The Clinic And It's Workers, Due To The Good Work Done At The Clinic.

7. A Systematic Comprehensive Chemical Health Record, Which Is Constantly Added To & Gives A Complete, Clear, Easy To Refer To, Picture Of The Problem, The Patient, His Background, Circumstances & Progress, With Special, Detailed Questionnaire/Records For ADD, Depression & Bipolar Disorder, Anxiety & Panic Disorders, Unresolved Psychosocial Trauma & Marital & Family Disharmony.

8. A Clear & Accurate Summary Of The Pre-existing Underlying Causes Of Drug Dependence In Each Case.

9. A Clear Multidisciplinary Management Plan, Discussed With And Accepted By The Patient.

10. A Full Range Of Medications, Quickly, Conveniently, Reliably & Safely Supplied, With Full Patient & Family Understanding Of The Effects & Side Effects Of These Medications.

11. EEG Biofeedback.

12. Full Information For Each Patient & Family On Everything To Do With The Causes, Nature & Treatment Of Addiction, Through Appropriate Teaching Aids, Handouts, Videos, Booklets & Websites, In Addition To the Usual Consultations With Healthcarers.

13. Assisted Detoxification Protocols That Provide A Solution Appropriate To The Needs Of Each Individual & Their Differing Addictions, Circumstances & Resources.

14. Frequent, Closed, Positive Focus, Positive Chemistry, Multi Strategy, Therapy Groups (Including Specialist Groups For ADD, Mood Disorders, Unresolved Psychosocial Trauma, Lack Of Direction & Purpose In Life And For Family & Marital Therapy).

15. Maintenance Pharmacotherapy as needed
    (a) Naltrexone or Buprenorphine
    (b) Serotonin Boosters (Cipramil, Efexor XR, Avanza, etc)
    (c) Mood Stabilisers (Epilim, Tegretol, Clonazepam, Lithium)
    (d) Stimulant Therapy (Ritalin, Dexamphetamine)

16. Professional Assistance in Social Recovery & Development of
    (a) A Stable, Satisfactory Home.
    (b) Friendships and of Family & Relationship Reconciliation & Development.
    (c) Education & Training.
    (d) Employment & Career and
    (e) Healthy, Pleasurable, Low Risk, Recreations.

EEG BIOFEEDBACK

Last year I attended a training programme in Brisbane run by a leading Australian EEG Biofeedback practitioner and the founder and principal of the main EEG Biofeedback company in the United States. It provided me with knowledge, understanding and skills which I had been hoping for, for over 40 years, since I was a medical student.

I think it is possible that EEG Biofeedback, over the next 20 years, will prove to be of great assistance in human progress. It is likely to have a very beneficial effect on the health of individuals and will be of great value in dealing with drug addiction and the drug trade, crime, learning problems and educational difficulties and such social problems as domestic violence and homelessness.

Your brain is the most important organ in your body. If your life is good that almost certainly means that you have a good brain. If you have serious problems, or your life is a nightmare, that is almost certainly due to having a malfunctioning brain. Whether your brain is structurally intact is not as important as whether its electrical currents and chemistry are flowing in a balanced and healthy way.

For many years we have known that abnormal brain waves are associated with epileptic convulsions. We have also known that these seizures can usually be stopped with anti-convulsant medications. What we should have realized many years ago, and should certainly know about by now, is that many forms of mental and social ill health and unhappiness, are due to, or associated with, unbalanced or abnormal electrical waves or currents and chemical flows in the brain. We now know that sleep disturbances, Attention Deficit Disorder, anxiety and depression, alcoholism, drug addiction, manic-depressive disorder, learning difficulties, chronic pain including migraine, compulsive gambling and disturbed emotions and behaviours, are due to or associated with abnormal brain waves and chemistry. We also now know that if we can give feed back to the brain indicating when it is functioning well and when it is functioning in an unhelpful way, it is usually capable of correcting itself. This is done with EEG Biofeedback.

In the early 1970's American scientists started to research EEG Biofeedback and made considerable progress. However because the results at that time were rather slow, and there were other exciting things that needed to be researched, research funds were diverted from EEG Biofeedback. Since the late 1980's, with much better and cheaper computers, much better software and renewed interest in this field, great progress has been made. The latest computers and software are capable of quickly detecting when someone's brainwaves are unbalanced or abnormal and when they are balanced and normal, and of feeding this information back to that person's brain. That person's brain can then learn to produce more and more of the balanced or normal electrical flows and less and less of the unbalanced or abnormal electrical flows.

Although 15 to 50 sessions of three-quarters of an hour on the Biofeedback computer program may be necessary to produce a cure, improvement may start within the first three or four treatments and great relief may sometimes be achieved within 10 to 20 treatments. However some problems are easier to correct than others.

The advantages of EEG Biofeedback are that there are not the side effects that often occur with medications and this treatment, when it is successful, and it usually is successful if properly used, is a cure rather than just a treatment that will have to go on long-term, as is usual with medications. It is true that some problems do not respond to this treatment and that some cases do not respond as well as others. Sometimes it is necessary to have booster treatments from time to time. It is a moderately time-consuming treatment and requires sophisticated, expensive equipment and is therefore moderately expensive. However compared to other forms of treatment, it can be more satisfactory and better value for money. Each treatment session usually costs between $50 and $100 depending on the individual healthcarer doing it.

HOW EEG BIOFEEDBACK IS DONE

In EEG Biofeedback you

(a) Put electrical activity sensing devices (electrodes) on the head of the person suffering from one of these health problems.

(b) Use leads to connect the electrodes to a computer, which then shows the person's brain waves (EEG or Electroencephalogram) on the screen and can print out a hard copy.

(c) Analyse the EEG for abnormalities.

(d) Get the patient to play games on an associated computer, not with their fingers and a button or a keyboard, but with their brain, through leads from the scalp, to the computer. Winning the game and rewards happen through scoring points and a beep, which occurs each time the patient gets their brainwaves balanced or in a normal pattern. The desire to improve their brainwaves or their brainwave patterns, is reinforced as they start to feel more comfortable and normal. Also as their family, friends and teachers start to congratulate them on their changed behaviour and reduced need for medication, and as they receive less discipline and punishment and get into fewer and fewer difficulties.

Cure may take 15 to 50 sessions of EEG Biofeedback (Neurofeedback), each lasting approximately three quarters of an hour. Of course, as with every other type of treatment, not everyone will be cured. However, if it does result in a cure, the various medications, which may have been a great help in getting the situation under control quickly to begin with, may be reduced, or phased out. Long term medications can be tedious, have side effects and don't resolve the problem completely or permanently. They may also be expensive.

THE HISTORY AND POTENTIAL FUTURE OF EEG BIOFEEDBACK

EEG Biofeedback has only recently become available in Australia but is going to become much more widely available. It will be expensive at first, but will probably be able to be streamlined and made much more efficient as the years go by, as with most new things. It will then become less expensive. However even now a course of EEG Biofeedback is likely to cost less than a few weeks on heroin, or the cost to the community of keeping someone in jail or in hospital for a few days, and there will be lasting and great benefits to the individual and the community, which heroin, jail or hospital don't usually yield.

EEG Biofeedback appears to have great potential to help in the **Heroin Detox Clinic** by correcting conditions such as ADD, depression, anxiety and insomnia, which cause people to start using heroin in the first place, and may cause them to relapse after being detoxed.

It is New Millennium technology which will be more effective in some people than the traditional medical/medication, psychological/psychotherapy approaches. It will also have much appeal for people familiar with computers and the internet, and those who "don't believe in" doctors, tablets and psychologists. However it is most likely to achieve its greatest effect as one component in a bundle of strategies which together have sufficient power to make real changes and produce results, that none of the individual strategies, old or new, can produce on their own. It will add an edge that will enable us to be successful with patients who are too difficult for us at present. It will enable us to be more productive and to be able to reach people who are beyond our present capabilities.

References
www.eegspectrum.com
www.snr-jnt.org

TOTAL REST (OBLIVION) THERAPY

Some unfortunate people find themselves in such a horrible internal state, or such terrible external circumstances, or both, that they cannot see any solution. They are in distress and despair and without hope. In desperation they may seek escape. They may take alcohol, valium, serepax, mogadon, cannabis etc and live in a sedated daze. They may take stimulants – nicotine, caffeine and speed and turn their life into a speedy affair, running away from their problems and pursuing varying objectives or overachievements. They may also use rohypnol, heroin, morphine, pethidine, amnesia, a nervous breakdown, or suicide to try to escape into oblivion.

The horrible internal states include mental disturbances such as depression, anxiety states, panic disorder, ADD, sexual conflict, obsessions, psychosis, alcoholism and chronic pain. The terrible external circumstances include family conflict, family or relationship breakdown, a bitter divorce with loss of contact with children, a death in the family, physical or sexual abuse, learning disabilities, bullying and other problems at school, problems in the workplace, financial disasters, horrific accidents, immigration and war experiences.

It is important that this condition or stage of seeking to escape into oblivion, be recognized in its sufferers generally, but especially in people who attend Heroin Clinics, or who seek treatment for heroin addiction. Heroin is the ultimate producer of oblivion. No superficial programme is going to help an oblivion seeking addict beat heroin and suicide may be an accidental or planned outcome. At least some of the internal and external problems must be discovered and resolved in order to reduce the load to tolerable levels. People don't go down because of just one problem – multiple problems, usually varied (genetic, chemical, brainwave, physical, mental, social) are needed to reduce a person to this state. Unless at least some of these problems are sorted out, detoxification from heroin is unlikely to succeed or to last.

If you recognize oblivion seeking in an addict it may be best to start by helping the patient to achieve oblivion in more efficient and less harmful or dangerous ways than the street drug, self medication methods they have been using. When they have rested and partly recovered and are stronger, they will be much better able to discover, face and resolve, at least some of their problems.

One technique I have used was to put such patients in hospital on substantial doses of amitriptyline, an older sedative type of antidepressant. For the first three days the patient would usually barely open their eyes, except to eat or drink. Then they would slowly and progressively wake up, as their tolerance for amitriptyline increased. After 3 or 4 days they were usually raring to get up and get on with sorting out their life, but I wouldn't let them get up till they were obviously much stronger and had resolved or formed strategies to resolve some of their problems. This plan is not often practicable now as few heroin addicts have private health insurance and public hospitals usually don't have beds for addicts in this condition.

Sometimes a family member is able to look after the patient at home. If so the patient should be encouraged to stay in bed and sleep most of the time, under heavy sedation day and night and to not even think about their problems. Falls and attempts at driving must be guarded against and the utmost care must be taken to avoid suicide, which is on the minds of many of these people. The safest way is to keep the patient heavily sedated and closely watched and have the pharmacist dispense only two or three day's medication every two or three days. Sometimes Webster Packs of medication are helpful. If the full bottles of medication are held by the carer, the patient may manipulate the carer into giving them too much, or may find where the medications are hidden and take an overdose whilst the carer is doing other things.

Tricyclic antidepressants such as amitriptyline are very useful for this treatment, but great care is needed as if a tricyclic overdose occurs, it may be fatal. Flunitrazepam (Rohypnol) can be tried and may be successful, but it is addictive and up to 30% of people who take it react adversely to it, trashing the house, becoming aggressive or violent, bashing other people or committing armed robbery and endangering themselves and others. Apart from or in combination with tricyclic antidepressants, Clonazepan 2mgms two to four times per day is usually the best medication. If they are not alcoholics, a beer, a glass of wine or some brandy in milk occasionally, may be a helpful addition. If they are ADHD sufferers some dexamphetamine or methylphenidate will be necessary to make sure they relax and sleep well. If they are narcotic addicts, they will need to be given sufficient buprenorphine to alleviate all withdrawal symptoms. If they are depressed, serotonin boosters will be helpful – non stimulant brands such as Efexor XR or cipramil are the best. The whole purpose of the exercise is to allow them to completely let go and rest, to be mothered like a child, to start to recover and regain some of their strength, composure and stability and to break the cycle of the ongoing destructive and dangerous drug rampage they have been on.

Whilst some oblivion seeking addicts will want to continue to pursue escape into limbo after their rest period, some will have broken the vicious cycle and become strong enough to want to go through Assisted Detox, to take Maintenance Therapy and to discover, face and deal with their Pre-existing Underlying Problems. Their lives will be transformed. If they are pushed to be detoxed without the rest period, recovery may not last and the danger of OD will be increased, if they go back onto narcotics again, with their tolerance reduced by a period of abstinence.

Heroin detoxification may be achieved during Oblivion Therapy using S.P.E.E.Q.E. detox.

H.M. female, 35 years.

H.M. hit our clinic like a cyclone. She was manic, severely depressed, extremely demanding and came or rang every day. She had very severe headaches, couldn't sleep and demanded immediate relief and solutions. The longer it got between sleeps, the worse she got. She was visiting hospitals and doctors every day, within a 25 km radius of her home. In the midst of all this she lost her transport when she drove her car (not insured) into the back of another car, when she looked down to make a phone call while she was driving. She has a multiply handicapped son who suffers from ADD and who demands a great deal of care and attention which he won't accept from his father. Her father died when she was three and her mother retreated into her shell, so that H.M. was raised by her elder sisters, who were still children themselves. Then her mother remarried, but the new stepfather sexually abused H.M., a matter which was hushed up by the family.

She is very much better now, but really should have had oblivion therapy to begin with. The nearest we could get to this was to give her overnight oblivion twice a week with 10mg of pericyazine, which sedated her well for 10-12 hours. It helped her a great deal, by breaking the vicious cycle she had been in.

NINE QUESTIONS FOR ADDICTS

1. What started me using drugs?
   What keeps me using drugs?

2. What am I and my life short of, deficient in?
   What am I normal in, or strong or gifted in?

3. Do I want to always be an addict and to always be a part of the drug world?

4. How did the people I know, who have got off and stayed off drugs, do it?
   What worked for them?
   Who helped them?

5. Will I need medicines?
   Where will I get them from?

6. What additional knowledge and understanding will I need?
   Where and how will I get that knowledge & understanding?

7. Are there any people or situations I need to get out of my life in order to be rid of drugs?

8. What counseling, therapy and support will I need?
   Where will I go to get it?

9. Is today the day to get started?
   What is the first step I will take?

SOME POINTS FOR HEROIN CLINIC HEALTHCARERS

There are some things which addicts value greatly and don't very often get. Examples are:

Non-judgmentalism. Addicts are continually judged by others and may be their own harshest judges. It helps them very greatly if they can tell you the worst, without fear of being judged verbally, or by your body language – the look on your face and the tones in your voice. More addicts have thanked me for being non judgmental than have thanked me for anything else. Non-judgmentalism is important to them in helping them to get everything out into the open and enabling them to start again.

Respect & Consideration. Addicts are usually treated like dirt and are seldom treated with respect or consideration. They usually don't respect themselves. It gives them a great lift and helps them succeed if you treat them with respect and consideration. Restoration of self- esteem is essential to recovery and it may start when someone is genuinely respectful and considerate towards them.

Kindness of the genuine, non-patronizing sort. Most addicts haven't experienced genuine, non-patronizing kindness, without conditions or a sting in its tail, for a long time. They need encouragement and hope, and that is what genuine, straightforward, non-patronizing, unconditional kindness does for them.

True Perception & Understanding of them and their individual situation is of great value to them. They are so used to being stereotyped and written off as junkies, as if they were the same as everyone else, that careful listening to and understanding of their individual situation, is a great encouragement to them.

Firmness. Some addicts have never had effective guidance, discipline, boundary setting or firmness in their life and this has allowed them to get into drugs. Sometimes you have to be firm, setting boundaries and sticking to them. This will often be appreciated, even if objected to at the time.

Non-Game Playing and Honesty. Many addicts have for a long time, moved in circles foreign to honesty and truth. They need to experience honesty, truth, openness and directness, in order to be able to discover or rediscover these things for themselves, as an essential part of living a satisfactory life. They are often thoroughly fed up with game playing and deception and are really refreshed by and grateful for some straightforward honesty.

Sexual Respect. Almost all female addicts have suffered sexual compromise, harassment or exploitation, and sometimes at the hand of healthcare professionals. Some feel that the only thing they have to offer is sex and may sometimes offer it. Some try to use their sexuality to get prescriptions, special treatment or a hold over you. If you have a high libido, perhaps you shouldn't work in the addiction field. What golden rules are you going to set for yourself, to protect your private relationships, integrity, self-respect and license to practice? If you are a male and can treat female addicts in a completely sexually respectful and non-sleazy manner it will usually be very greatly appreciated.

The Risk. If you have been an addict yourself, working with addicts may be a risky business. This is especially the case if you are a medical practitioner with the right to prescribe medications. The pressures involved may make it very dangerous. At times you may slip back to drugs yourself, or be persuaded to help someone out with drugs which it is illegal for you to prescribe for them. Knowledge, techniques and medicines now available, make it possible for healthcarer workers in the drug and alcohol field, to be effective in relieving suffering, restarting health and transforming lives in a way not often possible in other fields of healthcare. However these satisfactions may be outweighed by the risks and you need to care for yourself, as well as for your patients.

DUAL DIAGNOSIS OF SUBSTANCE ABUSE AND MENTAL DISORDERS: A CLINICAL STUDY

Wendy Jane Donaldson B.A. B. Psych   **Dr Neil Beck**

The need for dual diagnosis of substance abuse and mental disorders is becoming more and more evident through research worldwide (eg   Hattenschwiler, Ruesch, & Modestin, 2001; Hickie, Koschera, Davenport, Naismith, & Scott, 2001: Grella, Hser, Joshi, & Rounds-Hryant, 2001).   These reports suggest that mental disorders, such as anxiety (Regier, Narrow, Kaelber & Schatzberg, 1998), mood (Nunes, Deliyannides, Donovan, & McGrath, 1996), schizophrenia (Dixon, 1999), and personality disorders (Nadeau, Landry, & Racine, 1999), predominate in adults who abuse substances. Affective, Conduct, and Attention Deficit Disorders report most frequently for adolescents who abuse substances (Grella, et al, 2001).   A great concern is the increase in numbers of individuals who are seeking help for their substance abuse, and failing time and time again due to their undiagnosed mental disorder (Nunes et al, 1996). Attention Deficit Disorder (ADD), in particular, is a disorder that has received a great deal of attention in research as a common link to drug abuse for many years (eg Cocores, Davies, Mueler, & Gold 1987).   However, there has been controversy in diagnoses for many reasons.   The presumed recent over diagnosis, large quantities of prescribed amphetamines, and the denial of its existence, all contribute to the ADD sufferer being undiagnosed, due to Mental Health Workers' personal ignorance and this, therefore, often causes the patient to self medicate.   Also, it is only in recent times that it has been recognised that the sufferer may not 'grow out of' ADD by the time they reach adulthood.   Furthermore, the symptoms that are present may (for the child and the adult) be read as laziness, stupidity, or a lack of effort on the part of the sufferer.   This ill informed attitude sets the individual up to suffer the secondary symptoms of low self-esteem, depression, and a lack of self worth.   If the individual suffers enough pain they will often turn to the strongest painkiller available to them, heroin.   Heroin not only provides a relief from their chronically depressed feelings, but it also provides an environment that reinforces the belief that they are not a part of society as they are unable to function like most others.   However, it is not just the reluctance to seek underlying causes to an addiction in treatment, it is also the lack of knowledge and education provided to Mental Health Workers (Hall & Farrell, 1997).   Traditional treatment methods, that involve rapid detox, home detox, naltrexone, methadone, etc can be ineffective in the long run if the underlying causes of the addiction are not effectively treated, and will more often than not result in the patient repeatedly relapsing in the future. It is often reported by the patients attending this clinic, that it was the very next day after the completion of the treatments mentioned above, that they returned to their previously used drug. This strongly suggests that the reason that they began to use drugs in the first place, has not been effectively treated.

Research has reported wide variations in percentages of dual diagnoses, depending on the disorder and whether statistics were gathered from a population with mental disorder, or from a drug related population. For those with a life time diagnosis of schizophrenia (therefore not drug induced), 47% reported some form of drug abuse or dependence (Dixon, 1999). Regier, et al, (1998) studied a group of individuals who were all diagnosed with some categorisation of a mental disorder and found that about half of all the participants abused drugs in some form. Regier reported that of the adults with clinical depression 19% abused drugs, those with any mood disorder – 17%, and anxiety – 18% (Regier, et al, 1998). When participants were selected from populations with drug addictions the percentage for mental disorder increased. Personality disorder among clients in a drug detoxification treatment program rated around 50%, (Nadeau, et al, 1999). Of teenagers reporting drug abuse, 64% also reported as having at least one comorbid mental disorder, most frequently conduct disorder (Grella, et al, 2001). Although only a few studies have been reported here, similar findings are plentiful, and it is, therefore, suggested that when a population is made up of individuals who abuse drugs the prevalence of mental disorders is significantly high.

Filtration of effective help, however, is slow to reflect research findings (Hickie, et al, 2001). Clients at our clinic often report that doctors are all too quick to fulfil their requests for more prescriptions for addictive medications. If a patient reports to their doctor that they suffer from substance abuse and the doctor is willing to treat it, he is usually inclined to diagnose the problem to be treated as the addiction, and any other problems as secondary to the addiction (Hall & Farrell, 1997: Hickie, et al, 2001). Furthermore, even with mounting evidence that reveals the true nature of methadone (in regard to its capacity to reduce its user to a psychological and physical wreck) doctors still today, may encourage the heroin abuser to transfer over to it. This in itself suggests a lack of recognition for the link of a dual diagnosis by doctors and, therefore, the capacity to provide effective treatment that will benefit the client.

It is the intention of this report to support previous research findings with the statistics gathered from our clinic to further highlight the link between substance abuse and mental disorders. Also, to highlight the need for doctors to have the opportunity to provide addicts with appropriate medications, treatment, and access to other trained professional staff and facilities, in order to reduce the rate of relapse. GPs are presently operating in this field, with one arm tied behind their back.

Method

Participants
Participants were all drug dependant patients of some kind at our detoxification clinic in Victoria Park, Perth, Western Australia. The clinic serves the general population of southern Perth and attendance is entirely voluntary. The study comprised of 121 participants, with a minimum age of 17, maximum age of 54, and a mean age of 31 years. No statistics reported the difference between males and females.

Materials
All patients are required to fill out a Comprehensive Chemical Health Record (see List of Contents – Page 3) with the Clinical Assistant, who is trained to take detailed information from the client. This unpublished record was designed by Dr Neil Beck (2001) and allows for the recording of all demographic information; a detailed description of the patient's past and present drug use; personal characteristics that suggest neurobiological dysfunction; past or present traumas and/or stresses; family history; and any additional suspected underlying causes that led to their addiction. Information is recorded in either a qualitative manner or by circling suggested responses. All clients are asked to sign the record if they approve of their information (excluding their name) being used in research.

Results

SPSS was used to provide descriptive data on all 28 variables. The following descriptives are those of interest, refer to Appendix A for a comprehensive review.

Of the 121 participants, 32.2% have had confirmation by a psychiatrist for ADD, 28.9% are suspected, and are awaiting a psychiatrist's evaluation. Persistent, or above normal levels of anxiety or stress-related disorders was reported by 61.2% of the patients. 71.9% reported feeling abnormally sad or depressed (it is noted that this category does not distinguish between clinical depression, substance abuse related depression or high levels of sadness, which will be clarified in the discussion). Almost 10% were diagnosed with Bipolar Disorder; over 20% with Post Traumatic Stress Disorder; 22.3% with some kind of Personality Disorder; 13.2% with a Mood Disorder (not including Depression); and 7.4% with psychosis or schizophrenia.

Of the life events only 31.4% reported that their parents had divorced or separated. However, 55.4% reported that they were part of a dysfunctional family, and 14.9% were separated from their family for a long period of time that caused distress. 22.3% stated that they had immigrated, or that their parents had.

Drug related statistics showed that 82.6% were addicted to heroin, 73.6% abused amphetamines, 64.5% frequently used marijuana, 38% abused or were addicted to benzodiazapines, 36.4% had been on the methadone program, and 11.6% had abused prescription medications.

Discussion

The present study supports the link between substance abuse and mental disorders that has been reported in previous research (eg Hattenschwiler, Ruesch, & Modestin, 2001; Hickie, Koschera, Davenport, Naismith, & Scott, 2001; Grella, Hser, Joshi, & Rounds-Hryant, 2001). It suggests that individuals with mental disorders are at great risk of abusing drugs. This finding also highlights the importance of multiple screening for mental disorders when a patient presents with a substance addiction (Hickie, et al, 2001). The present study also pointed to the prevalence of social disorders, however the direction of the link is not clear.

Nunes, et al (1966) report on the necessity for professionals to be able to effectively treat all mental disorders when confronted by substance abuse. For example, it is mentioned that depression needs to be appropriately identified in those with addiction. Nunes suggests that depression can often confound successful detoxification, and encourages that the first stage of treatment should be to identify the depression and administer appropriate TCAs or SSRIs. Depression, or high levels of sadness often leaves the sufferer with the belief that there is little or no hope for a positive outcome. This will often make any effective progress slow, and difficult for the patient and the helper (Nunes, et al, 1996).

This finding strengthens the need for professionals working in drug related areas to be provided with the necessary funding to be able to provide effective treatment that takes into account more than just the addiction. These professionals need a body of trained professional staff to support all areas of abnormality requiring treatment. Treatment may include consultations from medically trained personnel and pharmacotherapy, all forms of counselling and referrals, and/or EEG Biofeedback treatment. EEG Biofeedback treatment is becoming a more acceptable form of treatment for individuals who are wishing to abstain completely from all drugs in the long run. This therapy is capable of treating many of the problems we see, ranging from sleeping problems to ADD, PTSD, depression and others.

In conclusion, it is suggested that a greater awareness and acceptance is needed by funding bodies, of the need to support the progress by detox clinics, towards providing all necessary treatment possibilities for substance abuse disorders, under one roof. It is recognised that there are few facilities within Australia (and possibly worldwide) that are willing to practice the holistic approach which we have chosen. Of great importance in the practical achievement of the diagnosis and treatment of these various mentally disordered people, (who have such difficulty in making, waiting for and keeping appointments), is the use of the 'shared consultation' technique which we have developed. This 'shared consultation' involves all patients coming together around a large consultation table as they arrive, without appointment, and the doctor attending to them one by one. During this time patients are encouraged to interact with the doctor and the patient being consulted. This environment provides support to others and the chance to share their experiences. Furthermore, the openness of the group encourages honesty with their issues, and the chance to face their situation in the presence of others. This speeds up the healing time as issues are confronted and dealt with on the spot.

It must be stated that the greatest impediment we have within our program, to successfully managing the patients who present to us, is getting psychiatric assessment of those suffering from ADD, and getting stimulant therapy for those who need it. It must also be said that the greatest triumphs we have in transforming the lives of clients with addictions, is when we discover that someone, who has been detoxed over and over again but keeps relapsing, suffers from ADD. With stimulant therapy the person and their life is totally changed. We would be dramatically improving our service if we were able to provide our clients with the opportunity to see a psychiatrist within our clinic. This would decrease the amount of time that a client would normally have to wait to see a psychiatrist, due to long waiting lists. Also, as stated before, it would remove the difficulty that is experienced by people with ADD, in making and keeping appointments. It would also reduce the substantial number who never make it to the psychiatrist and remain untreated and relapsing. It would also benefit our clients immensely if the option of EEG Biofeedback treatment was available. The addition of these aids would make our clinic more fully effective with this very substantial percentage of our patients who suffer from ADD. With the support of those who can make this possible, it is the belief of our clinic staff that we can make a great change in a positive direction towards reducing the high rate of relapse, amongst treated addicts.

References

Cocores, J. A., Davies, R. K., Mueller, P. S., & Gold, M. S (1987). Cocaine abuse and adult Attention Deficit Disorder. *Journal of Clinical Psychiatry*, 48, 376-37.

Dixon, L. (1999). Dual diagnosis of substance abuse in schizophrenia: prevalence and impact on outcomes. *Schizophrenia Research*, 35, s93-s100

Grella, C. E., Hser, Y., Joshi, V., & Rounds-Bryant,. J (2001). Drug treatment outcomes for adolescents with comorbid mental and substance use disorders. *The Journal of Nervous and Mental Disease,* 189(6), 384-391.

Hall, W., & Farrell, M. (1997). Comorbidity of mental disorders with substance misuse. *British Journal of Psychiatry*, 171, 4-5.

Hattenschwiler, J., Ruesch, P., & Modestin, J. (2001). Comparison of four groups of substance abusing in-patients with different psychiatric comorbidty. *Acta Psychiatric Scandinavia*, 104, 59-65

Hickie, I. B., Koschera, A., Davenport, T. A., Niasmith, T. A., & Scott, E. M. (2001). Comorbidity of common mental disorders and alcohol or other substance misuse in Australia general practice. *Medical Journal of America*, 175, s35-s37.

Kosten, T. R., Rounsaville, B. J., & Kleber, H. D. (1987). A 2.5 year follow-up of cocaine use among treated opioid addicts. *Archives of General Psychiatry*, 44, 281-284

Nadeau, L., Landry, M., & Racine, S. (1999). Prevalence of personality disorders among clients in treatment for addiction. *Canadian Journal of Psychiatry*, 44, 592-596.

Nunes, V. E., Deliyannides, D., Donavon, S., & McGrath, P. J. (1996). The management of treatment resistance in depressed patients with substance abuse disorders. *The Psychiatric Clinics of North America*, 19(2), 311-323.

Regier, D. A., Rae, D. S., Narrow, W. E., Kaelber, C.T., Schatzberg, A. F. (1998). Prevalence of anxiety disorders and their comorbidity with mood and addictive disorders. *British Journal of Psychiatry*, 173 (*suppl*, 34), 24-28.

APPENDIX A - FREQUENCIES

STATISTICS

Year born

N	Valid	120	
	Missing	1	
Mean		1970.35	Average age 31 years
Standard Deviation		7.89	
Variance		62.33	
Range		37	
Minimum		1947	Oldest 54 years
Maximum		1984	Youngest 17 years
Sum		8442	

FREQUENCY TABLE

A. SUBSTANCES ABUSED

Addiction to Heroin

		Frequency	Percent	Valid Percent	Cumulative Percent
Valid	not addicted	21	17.4	17.4	17.4
	addicted	100	82.6	82.6	100
	Total	121	100	100	

Amphetamine Abuse

		Frequency	Percent	Valid Percent	Cumulative Percent
Valid	not used	32	26.4	26.4	26.4
	used	89	73.6	73.6	100
	Total	121	100	100	

Frequent Marijuana Use

		Frequency	Percent	Valid Percent	Cumulative Percent
Valid	not used	43	35.5	35.5	35.5
	used	78	64.5	64.5	100
	Tota	121	100	100	

Abuse or Addicted to Benzodiazepines

	Frequency	Percent	Valid Percent	Cumulative Percent
Valid not abused	75	62	62	62
abused	46	38	38	100
Total	121	100	100	

Abuse or Addicted to Alcohol

	Frequency	Percent	Valid Percent	Cumulative Percent
Valid not abused	80	66.1	66.1	66.1
abused	41	33.9	33.9	100
Total	121	100	100	

Addicted to or Abuses Prescribed Medications

	Frequency	Percent	Valid Percent	Cumulative Percent
Valid not addicted	107	88.4	88.4	88.4
addicted	14	11.6	11.6	100
Total	121	100	100	

Is or has been on the Methadone Program

	Frequency	Percent	Valid Percent	Cumulative Percent
Valid not used	77	63.6	63.6	63.6
used	44	36.4	36.4	100
Total	121	100	100	

Time in Years that Patient has been Abusing Drugs

	Frequency	Percent	Valid Percent	Cumulative Percent
Valid less than 1 yr	4	3.3	3.8	3.8
1 – 2 years	11	9.1	10.4	14.2
3 – 5 years	20	16.5	18.9	33
6 – 8 years	22	18.2	20.8	53.8
8 or more yrs	49	40.5	46.2	100
Total	106	87.6	100	
Missing System	15	12.4		
Total 121	100			

Stage of their Treatment

		Frequency	Percent	Valid Percent	Cumulative Percent
Valid	just started	57	47.1	47.9	47.9
	out of danger	20	16.5	16.8	64.7
	mid way	37	30.6	31.1	95.8
	almost complete	2	1.7	1.7	97.5
	complete	3	2.5	2.5	100
	Total	119	98.3	100	
Missing	System	2	1.7		
Total	121	100			

B. CLINICAL DIAGNOSES

Depression

		Frequency	Percent	Valid Percent	Cumulative Percent
Valid	no	34	28.1	28.1	28.1
	yes	87	71.9	71.9	100
	Total	121	100	100	

Attention Deficit Disorder

		Frequency	Percent	Valid Percent	Cumulative Percent
Valid	no	47	38.8	38.8	38.8
	psychiatrist diagnosis	39	32.2	32.2	71
	clinic assumption awaiting psychiatrist confirmation	35	28.9	28.9	100
				Total ADD 61.1	
	Total	121	100	100	

Anxiety or High Levels of Stress

		Frequency	Percent	Valid Percent	Cumulative Percent
Valid	no	47	38.8	38.8	38.8
	yes	74	61.2	61.2	100
	Total	121	100	100	

Personality Disorder

	Frequency	Percent	Valid Percent	Cumulative Percent
Valid no	94	77.7	77.7	77.7
yes	27	22.3	22.3	100
Total	121	100	100	

Post Traumatic Stress Disorder

	Frequency	Percent	Valid Percent	Cumulative Percent
Valid no	95	78.5	78.5	78.5
yes	26	21.5	21.5	100
Total	121	100	100	

Mood Disorder

	Frequency	Percent	Valid Percent	Cumulative Percent
Valid no	105	86.8	86.8	86.8
yes	16	13.2	13.2	100
Total	121	100	100	

Bipolar Disorder

	Frequency	Percent	Valid Percent	Cumulative Percent
Valid no	109	90.1	90.1	90.1
yes	12	9.9	9.9	100
Total	121	100	100	

Psychosis or Schizophrenia

	Frequency	Percent	Valid Percent	Cumulative Percent
Valid no	112	92.6	92.6	92.6
yes	9	7.4	7.4	100
Total	121	100	100	

C. OTHER POSSIBLE CONTRIBUTORY FACTORS

Dysfunctional or Very Unloving Family

	Frequency	Percent	Valid Percent	Cumulative Percent
Valid no	54	44.6	44.6	44.6
yes	67	55.4	55.4	100
Total	121	100	100	

Parents Divorced or Separated

		Frequency	Percent	Valid Percent	Cumulative Percent
Valid	no	83	68.6	68.6	68.6
	yes	38	31.4	31.4	100
	Total	121	100	100	

MVA or Physical Injury Causing Pain

		Frequency	Percent	Valid Percent	Cumulative Percent
Valid	no	87	71.9	71.9	71.9
	yes	34	28.1	28.1	100
	Total	121	100	100	

Partner Is or Was Addicted

		Frequency	Percent	Valid Percent	Cumulative Percent
Valid	no	88	72.7	72.7	72.7
	yes	33	27.3	27.3	100
	Total	121	100	100	

Death of a Family Member or Loved One

		Frequency	Percent	Valid Percent	Cumulative Percent
Valid	no	90	74.4	74.4	74.4
	yes	31	25.6	25.6	100
	Total	121	100	100	

Parents or Client Immigrated

		Frequency	Percent	Valid Percent	Cumulative Percent
Valid	no	94	77.7	77.7	77.7
	yes	27	22.3	22.3	100
	Total	121	100	100	

Sexual Abuse

		Frequency	Percent	Valid Percent	Cumulative Percent
Valid	no	102	84.3	84.3	84.3
	yes	19	15.7	15.7	100
	Total	121	100	100	

Client was Separated from Family

		Frequency	Percent	Valid Percent	Cumulative Percent
Valid	no	103	85.1	85.1	85.1
	yes	18	14.9	14.9	100
	Total	121	100	100	

Domestic Violence

		Frequency	Percent	Valid Percent	Cumulative Percent
Valid	no	104	86	86	86
	yes	17	14	14	100
	Total	121	100	100	

If Client Received Counselling

		Frequency	Percent	Valid Percent	Cumulative Percent
Valid	no counselling	70	57.9	57.9	57.9
	counselling provided	51	42.1	42.1	100
	Total	121	100	100	

Z.Q. male, age 29

I attended Dr Beck's clinic with the hope of getting off heroin and speed. I was using $200 worth of heroin a day and one gram of speed per day and was quite a big dealer, which I needed to be to pay for my habits. Dr Beck found that over the years I had had head injuries, sleeplessness, anxiety, serious antisocial behaviour, compulsive gambling, suicidal thoughts and attempts, blood clots in the brain from bashing my head against a wall, and at one stage had been an alcoholic. I had been in jail six times and all my friends were drug users.

My father had been through war experiences and was extremely strict, almost brutal. One of my brothers was killed by electrocution when he was three and a half years old. The family broke up when my mother died. I had been married and had a son but lost him due to my jail periods. Dr Beck and Wendy thought that the main things leading to my addictions were my psychotic mother, the electrocution of my brother which caused terrible disturbances in the family, my harsh father, the loss of my son and ADD. I was put straight onto buprenorphine during the first consultation and didn't use illegal narcotics again. Dr Beck prescribed Epilim as first aid for the ADD but I didn't take it. The buprenorphine has been wonderful and I feel very much better and never crave other narcotics. However, I continue to use speed and Dr Beck has told me that I need to see a psychiatrist to look at the ADD possibility, as he feels that this is a very important underlying aspect of my condition. I lost my first referral to the psychiatrist, then missed my appointment twice, which Dr Beck tells me is common with ADD sufferers. I am now making every effort to get to see a psychiatrist as I really want to get off the speed.

Albany Highway
CHEMICAL HEALTH CENTRE

A SUBMISSION TO THE DRUG SUMMIT PERTH AUGUST 2001.

DR NEIL BECK
Provider No: 187242H
A.B.N. No: 66 900 952 705

PROGRESS IS SLOW IN ADDICTION MEDICINE.

There are five types of medication which, in varying combinations and sequences, provide the most effective pharmacotherapy for most people suffering from narcotic addiction. (Buprenorphine, Serotonin Boosters, Valproate, Dexamphetamine and Naltrexone) One of these types of medication has been available for 10 years and the others have been available for 20 to 40 years. Yet we still don't, or aren't allowed, to make optimal use of these medications.

Western medicine still largely fails to recognize the importance in the treatment of drug and alcohol addiction, of diagnosing and treating the Pre-existing Underlying Problems in each individual case, even though in most other fields of medicine this has been standard practice for many years. In other fields of medicine we want to know what the etiology was, but in addictions we don't seem to bother. Each addiction was always preceded by Underlying Problems. These problems must be discovered and dealt with in every case, if treatment of the addiction is to be truly successful, and relapse is to be avoided.

Western medicine still has not recognized that the largest, most easily diagnosed and most readily treated group of people addicted to illicit drugs, are the undiagnosed ADD sufferers. Rapid progress could be made with the whole drug problem, at very limited additional cost to begin with and great savings later, if this obvious fact was recognized.

Untold unnecessary suffering has been going on in Western Australia for more than 17 years, since Dr Pat Cranley was stopped from using Buprenorphine in 1984, and they grew the methadone program instead. It is obvious that Buprenorphine is a very safe, painless, easy, effective, quick, and economical pharmacotherapy for narcotic addiction. Buprenorphine has already been safely and extensively used in Australia since the early eighties, for pain. It was an S4 drug and could therefore be prescribed without restriction by any WA doctor. It has been very widely and successfully used to treat narcotic addiction in France since 1995. Any doctor in the U.K. can use it, to treat narcotic addiction. It was approved by Government in early 2001 for use by Primary Care doctors in the U.S.A., for the treatment of narcotic addiction although final approval from the FDA may not yet be through. Now after more than 17 years, our W.A. policy makers and enforcers have only just started to allow us to use Buprenorphine again, in the treatment of narcotic addiction. But still with unnecessary controls and restrictions, which significantly reduce it's usefulness and slow our progress, with very unfortunate consequences for addicted members of our community, as well as for our general community safety and quality of life.

WHEN THERE IS A SAFE EFFECTIVE NEW MEDICINE, WHY USE A REALLY NASTY, OLD, OUT OF DATE MEDICINE ?

Methadone is such a nasty alternative to Buprenorphine, with so many side effects and shortcomings. It was discovered in Germany in 1938 and is an outdated drug that should have been replaced by Buprenorphine when Buprenorphine first became available in the early eighties. Doctors and clinics that put patients onto Methadone in 2001 may yet in some cases be sued for the suffering and damage it often causes. As it is more and more widely realised that the great majority of addicts primarily have a sickness or have been traumatized, rather than primarily being moral failures, it will also be more widely realised that, like other sick people, they have rights and are entitled to prompt effective humane treatment. The more widely the results of treatment with Buprenorphine become known, the less defensible the current use of Methadone will be and the more accountable mistaken and sluggish authorities will become for what has happened over the past 17 years and is still happening. Do the Drug and Alcohol authorities really need to wait till the lawyers start to attack them, before they make progress and get their act together? I have one patient who is at present gearing up to sue the authorities. He appears to have a strong case, although it is a bit of a David and Goliath scenario.

MOST ADDICTS HAVE DONE NOTHING TO DESERVE WHAT IS HAPPENING (OR NOT HAPPENING) TO THEM, OR THE MENTALITY OF THE PEOPLE WHO CONTROL THEIR MANAGEMENT.

The majority of addicts are no more to blame for their situation than is someone who has asthma, heart disease, cancer or multiple injuries from a motor vehicle accident in which they were not the driver. They don't deserve to be treated with contempt and left to wait and wait and suffer and rot, whilst experienced, commonsense healthcarers, who don't need exhaustive trials in order to see what needs to be done, or to be policed in order to be made "safe", are held back from getting the job done, by "help" and rules and regulations from Next Step and the Health Department.

Although they both appeared to make some mistakes, ended up at loggerheads with the authorities and had to appear before the Medical Board, at least one had the feeling that Dr. Pat Cranley and Dr. George O'Neil were very bright lateral thinking human beings, who cared a lot, and who were getting on with the job of finding more expeditious means for treating addicts, to whom they were close and with whom they personally worked, face to face, on a daily basis. I sometimes get a different feeling in my contacts with some of the Drug and Alcohol healthcare professionals and officials, who occupy senior positions.

If you fell down a well and were wet, freezing and in danger of drowning, some of these people would say to you "I can't throw you this rope that I have here in my hand, until we have done extensive studies on it. We assume that all ropes are going to break, until exhaustive studies have proved otherwise, even if other people have been using these ropes for many years. We do not understand or trust common sense – in fact we despise it. Our rope studies will only take 2 years, but we can't start until we have had 3 years (or 17 years) to think about it, hold committee meetings, decide how the studies should be carried out and apply for research grants. We are sorry that in the meantime we have to leave you down the well, but it is for your own protection. We have to be terribly careful not to do anyone any harm, even if this makes our progress so slow that some people might think we are going backwards. We also have to be very active in preventing the risk that other doctors, using their own intelligence and initiative, may do some harm. We don't really understand their way of thinking and working and we are sorry that we get in their way and retard their progress. But we must try to make sure that what they do is risk free, even though with drugs and addiction, doing nothing or slowing things down, leads to suffering, disease and deaths. We believe everything should be centrally controlled, and we are the ones who should have that control."

These experts who control what we can and can't do for our addict patients, remind me of a farmhand I once had working for me. We had a small bulldozer on the farm and the farmhand didn't want anyone except himself to be allowed to operate the bulldozer. He used to tell us about all the things that could go wrong with a bulldozer and then get on and drive it, in a way that made driving it look terribly complicated and difficult. He didn't get the job done, so eventually we had to call his bluff and let others do some of the driving. It turned out that other people could drive the bulldozer perfectly well and the job got done.

THE GOOD NEWS AND THE BAD NEWS IN 2001.

The good news in the year 2001 is that we now have all the tools and techniques needed to beat drugs and the underlying factors that lead to addiction, in the vast majority of cases. Progress and fine tuning will naturally occur and further breakthroughs would be very welcome. Of course there is a great need for far wider recognition, understanding, availability and freedom to use what we have already got and what we already know. But no more major technical breakthroughs are necessary before we can break the back of the drug problem and the misery, disease and cost it causes our people and our communities. I know I will lose credibility in the short term for making this statement, but it is very important that the general community should know where we are and not be bluffed by the bulldozer drivers. (I am willing to wait for vindication down the track). We don't even need more government money than what we can already get through bulkbilling Medicare, provided there is some funding for psychologist and social worker back up.

The bad news is that we may not be allowed to get on with the job. Too much State Government money is being wasted by the authorities getting in our way and "helping" us. Will we be encouraged and supported, or will we be restricted, obstructed, and slowed down with paperwork and having to make applications for authority to prescribe medications, to people who know the rules, but who are quite out of touch with and don't know or understand the widely differing patients and their greatly varying circumstances, that we are treating.

IMMEDIATE, TAILOR MADE, COMMONSENSE, ON THE SPOT, MEDICAL HELP IS ESSENTIAL FOR SUCCESS WITH ADDICTS.

When an addict comes in and says they want to get off heroin "now", and are ready to fight and suffer in order to achieve this, that is the moment at which we need to be able to give immediate, effective, unfettered, tailor made relief and treatment. Until that moment comes, there is little we can do for an addict. Once that moment arrives, there is no time to be wasted. When addicts are hot they are hot, but they don't often stay on the boil for very long, because of the nature of their illnesses, their pressing needs and circumstances, and their personality types. If treatment is delayed for half, one, two or three days, until we have done the paperwork and got permission to prescribe what was needed at the time that the patient first came in, it is often too late. The addict may by then, in desperation, have had to find relief elsewhere and be stuck back in the world of fast moving dealers and crime. Or in frustration and disgust at the "holier than thou" indifference and sluggishness of our response to their severe suffering and urgent needs, the addict may have given up hope and turned their backs on us and our clinics and institutions. The next time they reach a similar turning point in their lives, the whole frustrating cycle may well be repeated. In the meantime they may have been in jail, got Hep C or lost their family. An addict wanting to get off heroin is at least as much of a medical emergency as appendicitis, broken bones or pneumonia and, as with those conditions, the problem shouldn't be left till the next day or for a week or two for assessment and treatment.

BRAINWASHING AND INTIMIDATION BY UNWISE, POWER HUNGRY, CONTROL FREAKS.

The rules introduced in Western Australia in 1984, to deal with the Cranley/ Buprenorphine "problem", made and still make it even more of a sin for a doctor to give Buprenorphine to an addict, than to give morphine to an addict, without Health Department approval, even though the value and safety of Buprenorphine is now recognized worldwide. The present plan in WA seems to be that only a few doctors will be allowed to prescribe Buprenorphine for addicts, and those doctors will have to pass an exam set by Next Step. Recently, 2 days after a newspaper article about a Heath Department/Next Step bungle with one of my patients, I was advised that I had failed the examination which I needed to pass in order to be allowed to continue to prescribe Buprenorphine. I have now been prescribing Buprenorphine for well over a year, with great success and no problems. I nearly didn't do the exam as I felt that I would fail it unless I gave answers which I didn't believe were correct, but which were the answers that the authorities wanted to hear, based on what other doctors, who agree they are also learning, have said. Also the exam was partly a brainwashing exercise, which I resented. But they had put those of us who already had our own experience with Buprenorphine, in a lose/lose situation. I was certain to lose if I didn't do the exam so I did it as best I could. Now one doctor, who was a key opponent of Buprenorphine and who favoured methadone in 1984, and an administrative doctor who does not have clinical responsibilities or current clinical experience, are hinting that by the end of July I may not be allowed to continue to prescribe Buprenorphine. My position shows some progress on Dr Cranley's position in 1984, but not a lot. Addiction Medicine moves very slowly.

They recently jokingly told me that nearly all private doctors who get involved in Addiction Medicine, end up before the Medical Board. That just might have been meant to put me off, or it may have been a friendly piece of good advice, but I am not a person who is very easily put off. However the frustrations of trying to make progress in Addiction Medicine in Perth, are certainly sufficient to put some doctors off and to drive some other doctors, who care about patient health and suffering, general community safety and quality of life, and the welfare of their children and grandchildren, to sometimes think about how to get out of touch rules and regulations changed. I personally, because of family responsibilities, wouldn't break the law to try to help a patient, but can understand why some doctors would and do.

Could the authorities hope to brainwash and humiliate private practise solution seekers into submission with their exam, and their capacity to fail and exclude us, by deciding which answers are correct and which are incorrect in a field where there are still genuine differences of opinion? I personally don't get brainwashed or humiliated very easily. Common sense, not exams, was always my strength. I have failed exams before and still come through. And I am in good company – they also failed Dr Pat Cranley, who was smart enough to spot the fantastic possibilities of Buprenorphine 18 years ago, when it was just another unrestricted S4 painkiller, which any doctor could prescribe. Both Pat and I were given 7 marks out of 15 and so failed the exam. I wonder what mark they will give us next time? Dr George O'Neil has not yet found time in his busy program, to do their exam and why should he if they are only going to fail him? I wonder what mark they will decide to give him and if he doesn't find the time to do the exam, will it mean that Next Step and the Health Department will stop him using Buprenorphine? I think George, Pat and I will be able to survive their power games and brainwashing between us, if necessary with public and media support.

HISTORY WILL JUDGE US.

In the end I think history will judge us mainly for failing to recognize the importance of discovering and addressing precisely, the Pre-existing Underlying Problems in each individual person suffering from an addiction; and for putting small minded control orientated people with a proven record of making bad decisions, rather than smart, wise people with open, lateral thinking minds, in charge of such an important area as substance abuse.

It is time for us to focus on discovering and treating the underlying causes in each case of addiction. Is it also time for us to make a fresh start, by leaving behind those Next Step/Health Department officials who have the type of mentality that chose Methadone over Buprenorphine in 1984 and that tries to exert unnecessary beaurocratic control of the coalface workers, in 2001. Let us make our decisions on the basis of the needs of cold, hungry, homeless people tortured by disturbed chemistry, and the families and communities they cause havoc in, rather than worrying too much about preserving the jobs of some people who have 3 meals a day, sleep in warm beds in nice suburbs and don't really know what is going on, and who many addicts and families feel have let them down very badly.

Many people who read this Submission will be offended by it. I can understand people feeling that way and genuinely regret that I believe it is necessary to cause this distress in order to get things changed. I can assure readers that what I have written arises directly out of everyday contact with real life people, in real life situations and the need, for everyone's sake, to make progress with the terrible problem of addiction and it's underlying causes. A less blunt statement of the situation is likely to be too easily glossed over and forgotten by politicians and authorities, with nothing being done.

The good news is that I think we may be on the verge of making serious progress with problems that have been the scourge of many people and families in most communities, for hundreds of years.

A SIMPLE OVERVIEW OF HOW WE HUMAN BEINGS FUNCTION & SOME OF THE WAYS IN WHICH WE MAY MALFUNCTION

1. **We function physiologically** – we breath air in and out, getting oxygen in and expelling carbon dioxide. Our heart beats and pumps blood to all parts of our body. We contract and relax our muscles to allow us to move and to do things.

2. **We have sensory function** – we see with our eyes, we hear with our ears, we touch and smell and taste.

3. **We function emotionally** – we respond to internal and external things with happiness, joy, love, surprise, sadness, fear, anger, guilt etc.

4. **We have intellectual function** – we see, hear and feel in our mind, as well as calculating and deciding things in our mind. In our mind we can focus on the past, the present or the future (remember, think or imagine).

5. **We function chemically** – we produce hundreds or thousands of different chemicals in our body and our brain, in addition to all the chemicals we eat, drink, smoke, or inject. We use, store, break down and excrete these chemicals. These chemicals underlie and enable our physiological, sensory, emotional and intellectual functioning, our actions, perceptions, mood, and pace. Some of our chemistry is "positive" – when we produce or take in some chemicals in appropriate amounts, we feel good and function well. Some of our chemistry is "negative" - when we produce or take in some, or too much, or not enough, of some chemicals, we feel bad and function poorly.

6. **We function socially** – we communicate, act and react, love and fight, form relationships, families, groups, communities and nations.

7. **We function spiritually** –

8. **Our lives are determined largely** – by the genes within us, which came from our two parents and four grandparents; major happy and unhappy events and circumstances in the past, which were strong enough to have an enduring effect on our structure and functioning; our present circumstances and our perception of these circumstances; and our beliefs about our future prospects.

EACH OF THESE TYPES OF FUNCTIONING CAN GO WRONG IF WE

1. Inherit too many abnormal genes.

2. Suffer physical injury or disease.

3. Have chemical deficiencies, excesses, or allergies, leading to abnormal chemistry.

4. Experience psychological pressures, traumas or disasters, especially if there are several, one on top of the other.

5. Experience social pressures, traumas or disasters, especially if several occur one, after another, so that before one is resolved another occurs.

6. Have faulty belief systems.

THINGS FUNCTION WELL IF WE

1. Have mostly normal genes.

2. Have most of our basic needs met, most of the time.

3. Don't suffer too many injuries, chemical deficiencies excesses or allergies, or psychological traumas or pressures and

4. Recover from each of our social pressures, traumas or disasters, before the next one hits us.

5. Have realistic belief systems.

6. Have positive chemistry and are optimistic.

SOMETIMES WE NEED TO

1. Reassess our situation and ourselves.

2. Gain new knowledge or

3. Skills

4. Do repair work

5. Make changes or

6. Get help

If we are not functioning to our satisfaction, or are running into too much trouble with the people and the world around us.

THE HUMAN FUNCTION CYCLE or
THE DETECTION DECISION ACTION CYCLE

With our senses we see, hear, feel, taste, smell – and –

In our brain we remember, think or imagine
(see, hear, feel, taste, smell in our mind).

Chemical production occurs (neurotransmitters, hormones etc) in response to our sensations and thoughts. These chemicals flow through our body transmitting messages and activating or suppressing our various functions and parts.

Electrical Currents flow throughout our brain, from one part to another, transmitting messages and activating or inhibiting various parts and functions. There are short frequency and long frequency brain waves.

We may then talk with others and make conscious or unconscious decisions as a result of these sensations and thoughts. We then do or don't do things as a result of our decisions.

This sequence of events may be called **The Detection, Decision, Action Cycle.**

Most of our day we are looking, listening, feeling, thinking, deciding, talking, doing. Most of us can't do more than two to four of these things well at once. For various reasons some people do too much of some of these things and therefore can't do as much of the other things as they may need to be doing, in order to live a satisfactory life. For example, some people don't see the things around them because they are so occupied with seeing things in their head – that is they think too much. If you have a strong habit of visualizing things in your head whilst talking about them at the same time, then you will not be able to also notice whether the people you think you are communicating with, are listening and interested, or are bored and have stopped listening. Some people talk and do so much that they don't hear, think or feel much.

Healthy people are balanced and flexible – they automatically carry out the functions in the **Detection, Decision, Action Cycle** that are most needed and helpful at the time. People who are in trouble in their life are usually unbalanced and inflexible in their **Detection, Decision, Action Cycle** habits. They habitually concentrate excessive effort or resources in some areas and then fall short in others. They may be very visual and be very focused on whatever there is to be seen, but not hear or feel much. Or they may always be very busy, active people who can't, won't or don't think or plan and have difficulty with decision making.

It is possible to observe what the problems are with people who don't function well and who are consequently in distress and cause problems for those around them. It is then possible to greatly improve their quality of life and the quality of life of those around them, by correcting their imbalances, freeing up their rigidities and strengthening their weak areas. Many addicts make snap judgements and are very rigid in their beliefs. They may need therapy to overcome these dysfunctions – group therapy is usually the most effective way to do this. In group therapy you experience how others see, feel and think and this gives you new options to choose from.

SOME COMMON HUMAN MALFUNCTIONS

Sensing Too Much, Sensing Too Little

Feeling Too Much, Feeling Too Little

Thinking Too Much, Thinking Too Little

Talking Too Much, Talking Too Little

Doing Too Much, Doing Too Little

Too Internally Focused and Too Insensitive to What Is Going On Externally

Too Externally Focused and Oblivious To What Is Going On Internally

Too Focused On The Past

Too Focused On The Future

1. We may **do too much** of some things in the **Detection Decision Action Cycle** and therefore not be able to do enough of other things, as we can usually only do 2 to 4 things in the Cycle at once. Or we may **not do enough** of some things in the Cycle and therefore end up doing too much of other things, because of all the time and energy we have left over.

   (a) We may be too sensory/sensual, too much in our senses, always seeing, listening, feeling, tasting and not thinking, communicating or doing enough.

   (b) We may be always thinking (seeing, hearing and feeling things in our head), living in our head, and failing to see, hear and feel what is going on around us. Our focusing span is not sufficient to cover everything and the more we do of one, the less we can do of the others.

   (c) We may remember too much, living in the past, often dwelling on the unhappy things from the past. This activates our negative chemistry and we feel bad, perhaps feeling helpless or despairing and disempowered, or badly or unfairly treated. We may imagine too much, always speculating about the future, or far away places, and often worrying about bad things that might (but probably won't) happen in the future. This further activates our negative chemistry. We may not think enough about the present, or not spend enough time seeing, hearing and feeling what is going on around us and in us now, and not doing things now, so that we don't live the most important part of our life, which is here and now.

(d) We may talk too much, or do too much, not allowing ourselves to do enough sensing, thinking, learning, decision making and planning.

(e) We may disturb our function through poor nutrition and inadequate exercise, rest and recreation, resulting in disturbed chemistry, fatigue and mental and physical weakness. Our genetic makeup and our bodies and chemistry, inherited from thousands of generations of ancestors, is based on natural high fibre foods and a physically active life style in the fresh air and sunlight, but we may live on processed, refined foods with unnatural additives, and live a sedentary lifestyle, with little exercise, in a polluted atmosphere with little sunlight.

(f) We may disrupt our natural chemistry, and thus our natural functioning, with foreign chemicals that we eat, drink, inhale or inject. If we have genetic problems, especially chemical problems or physical, mental or social health problems, we may take chemicals to help the distress, pain or weaknesses they cause, but chemicals are sometimes blunt instruments that may have undesirable side effects. We need to know what the benefits from these chemicals are going to cost us in undesirable side effects and after effects, before we start them, especially if they cause dependency or addiction.

We may use chemicals to augment sensations, thoughts, physical strength, performance and endurance, to try to be "larger than life", but this usually backfires and costs us more in the end, than we gain in the short term. However if our problems are very severe and cause us to hurt badly enough, or we are weak and immature, we may seek immediate relief and have a "to hell with the future" attitude. We may then put off the hell for a while, but when we get to it, if it is narcotics we have resorted to, the hell can be pretty bad. Fortunately modern medicine and therapy can now help most people avoid or fight their way through this stage.

ADD or ATTENTION DEFICIT DISORDER.

One of the common disturbing forms of Human Malfunction is ADD or Attention Deficit Disorder. It could more helpfully be called Attention/Focusing/Activity/ Impulsivity/Time Awareness, Malfunction and Suffering.

In my practice I have found ADD to be the commonest cause of heroin addiction. Heroin blanks out the suffering caused by the malfunctions and distress of ADD, but then causes other terrible problems.

ADD is a genetically determined chemical disorder which is aggravated by stress and misfortunes. It also snowballs because of the effects of the malfunctioning. It is often wrongly put down to poor parenting and misbehaviour, further aggravating the problem through guilt, loss of self esteem and unjust blame. The suffering caused can be very severe, both for the patient and his family and especially if there is more than one ADD sufferer in the family, as there often is.

The actual mechanism of ADD is ultimately chemical in nature and is thought to be due to faulty regulation of the supply of the brain chemicals Serotonin, Dopamine, Adrenaline and Noradrenaline. This leads to faulty Attention/Focusing. Activity and Drive is usually excessive but may be deficient. Responses and Decisions are often very rapid, impulsive or knee jerk in nature and are therefore often unhelpful. Time Awareness is often a serious problem for ADD sufferers. Five minutes waiting may seem like forever to these people, whilst at other times they may become focused on some activity for hours and hours and not notice the time going by, or that they haven't eaten or slept and have missed appointments and other duties.

ADD leads to poor learning capabilities, poor work and career prospects, family and relationship stresses, unhappiness - at times extreme - and a strong tendency to substance abuse, as a form of desperate but unhelpful self medication.

The treatment includes medicines (Epilim, Efexor XR, Doxepin, Dexamphetamine and Ritalin), educational assessment and special catch up education, counselling, development of work skills, career and relationships and recognition and utilization of the special abilities and talents ADD sufferers often have.